# NECESSARY
# TOUGHNESS

# NECESSARY TOUGHNESS

*Facing Defenses and Diabetes*

## By Jonathan Hayes
### with Robert L. Briggs

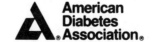

American
Diabetes
Association

This book was made possible in part by
a grant from Miles Inc., Diagnostics Division,
marketer of the
GLUCOMETER ELITE™
Diabetes Care System.


The American Diabetes Association and
the co-authors would like to thank
Miles Inc.,
Diagnostics Division
for its generous support of this project
and its ongoing service to the
diabetes community.

American Diabetes Association
1660 Duke Street
Alexandria, Virginia   22314

Printed in the United States of America
98  97  96  95  94  93     5  4  3  2  1

*Library of Congress Cataloging-in-Publications Data*

Hayes, Jonathan, 1962-
          Necessary toughness:  facing defenses and diabetes / by
Jonathan Hayes with Robert L. Briggs


          1. Hayes, Jonathan, 1962-     . 2. Football players--United
States--Biography.        3. Diabetics--United States--Biography.
I. Briggs, Robert L., 1956-     . II. Title.
GV939.H345A3 1993     796.332'092--dc20 [B]        93-11172
ISBN 0-945448-30-9

# DEDICATION

I would like to thank my mother and father for all the strength and guidance they have given me and for being my number one fans—I'm their number one fan, too.

— JH

# CONTENTS

# PREFACE

At age 21, just as I was stepping out of adolescence through the door of adulthood, I learned that diabetes was to be a part of my future.

This book is an attempt to help remind those of you with diabetes--more than 13 million Americans--that you have a serious disease and that you must never underestimate the threat it presents to your body. But, at the same time, I want you to know that if you are willing to pay the price for managing your disease properly, you can continue to live a satisfying life and reach for your dreams.

Some of you do not have diabetes. This book is for you as well. It is not only about a pro football player facing the challenges of managing a chronic disease; it is about a person confronted with serious adversity. Mine has taken the shape of type I diabetes. Yours may take another form.

As I have tackled my adversity, I have learned about myself, about people, and about what's valuable in life. My hope is that my story will encourage you to build success with whatever gifts you have been given. My intent is to help propel you forward, beyond the obstacles that threaten to derail your dreams.

Several years have transpired between the writing of this book and the accounts described. To help tell the story, I have recreated some dialogue. The material contained within quotes is an effort at capturing the essence of a conversation's content and may not reflect the actual words spoken.

The volunteers and staff of the American Diabetes Association, Missouri Affiliate, Inc., deserve much credit for this project. In 1991, I listened to their proposal about this book and concluded that perhaps it could help other people if I were to tell my story. We started in, and they have helped us along the way.

I also want to thank many people who helped with the development of this project. Linda Larson, the nurse who first spoke to me about diabetes management at the University of Iowa Hospital, helped by sending me a file full of data regarding my initial diagnosis and treatment. Not only did Linda encourage me during the initial period following my diagnosis, but I consider her a friend.

Brenda Boatright, who works in the public relations office of the Kansas City Chiefs, helped assemble various pieces of information that we needed. Hank Young allowed us to use the two photographs that appear on the front and back covers, and he helped coordinate the cover design. Bob Gretz, a Kansas City area sportswriter and broadcaster, helped review the manuscript and strengthen key portions of the story.

I certainly want to thank the Miles Inc., Diagnostics Division, for generous help in underwriting some of the costs of publishing this book.

— JH

# NECESSARY
# TOUGHNESS

# CHAPTER
### 1

# COLLEGE
# CRISIS

In many ways, my life may be dramatically different from yours. My life started out with a few God-given talents that can open a door to opportunity. Because I was born into a healthy home where hard work and tough inner discipline was encouraged, my physical skills were mixed with an unquenchable motivation to excel. The result has been an opportunity to join an elite fraternity of men who play in the National Football League.

First, I became one of the 10 percent of high school football players who make the jump to the college level. Then in 1985, I became the 42nd of the 334 college football players drafted by the 28 National Football League teams when the Kansas City Chiefs selected me in the second round.

I managed to survive that first training camp to become one of the 10% of college players who make the jump to the professional level, and I have been able to maintain steady performance over the years at tight end.

While a career in the National Football League exacts a great price in terms of wear and tear on a body, it also carries with it benefits. But don't let the glamour connected with professional sports confuse you. In many ways, my life is not at all different from yours. As you read my story, you'll see for instance that life in the NFL provides no defense against many kinds of adversity that can strike a person. It provided me no defense for the assault from a disease like diabetes.

If you have diabetes and take insulin, you and I both have to search every day for a spot on our bodies that's not already sore where we can give ourselves a shot. We both have to prick a finger several times a day to check the sugar level in our blood. We both have to pay careful attention to cuts and scratches to make sure they heal properly. When our friends head out to have some fun, we both have to make sure we have a snack with us. When we order dinner at a restaurant, we both have to think through the ingredients of each dish and anticipate the result on our sugar levels. No matter how successful my football career becomes, my day-to-day tasks to manage diabetes are the same as yours. Even if my team wins the Super Bowl, I earn All-Pro honors, and get inducted into the Hall of Fame, I'll still have to get up every morning and take that shot of insulin that keeps me healthy.

Diabetes was not a dominant issue in my family. The only connection I knew of was one cousin who was diagnosed when he was young. But that limited exposure to the disease in no way prepared me for its attack on my seemingly invincible body.

Not a moment goes by when I can forget that I have diabetes. Managing this disease is a minute-by-minute, hour-by-hour job. It's not a matter of stopping in to see my doctor every month or so. The doctor, nurses, and my dietitian, all play key roles in adjusting insulin dosages, watching for complications, and monitoring my overall health. But they aren't there in the morning when I get up to check my blood. I have to pull the monitor out myself, stick my already-sore finger yet another time, place a drop of blood on a test strip, and see what my sugar level is. No one is there to do it for me. I have to serve as the doctor of my own body.

At first, like most people, I wanted to ignore the disease. I wanted it to just go away. Managing diabetes had not been part of my plan, and I wanted nothing to do with writing a new script for my life. But, as anyone with diabetes can tell you, ignoring the disease doesn't make it disappear.

Finally, I learned that this is something that required far more than casual care. I would have to change the way I lived my life. Fortunately, I had some good building blocks to start with.

The explanation for my ability to face diabetes begins with my family. My grandparents taught my parents about hard work and what is important in life. My parents in turn laid a good foundation for my brothers and me. The work ethic I observed at home carried over onto the athletic field and into the weight room. My physical strength is no accident. My muscle tone is a result of hours, weeks, months, and years of dedicated toil in the weight room. My accomplishments on the field point back to a confidence and an internal drive to excel that emerged from my home life.

Life in my home was disciplined. I learned self-control and an ordered lifestyle. I developed an inner strength from a healthy family upbringing that left me a step ahead when confronted with the lifestyle changes required to properly manage diabetes.

When a nurse told me I would have to change my eating habits, it wasn't revolutionary because I had already incorporated a good dose of discipline into my everyday life. I could make the changes without too much anguish.

She also told me that exercise could be an important component in controlling diabetes. Again, a disciplined approach to exercise required no adjustment. I had rarely missed a day in several years of pushing myself hard through a workout, either lifting weights, riding a stationary bike, jogging, or, of course, exerting myself through a football practice or game. The trick for me was to learn when to let up and when to push, how to regulate the exercise to have the desired effect on my blood sugar level.

Like anyone, sometimes my motivation dips a bit. I'll be tempted to let up on my regimen. For instance, if a bunch of teammates go out to eat, they often start the meal with a drink. I can't. I have to get something to eat first. So when the waiter starts around the table, the first guy orders a drink, second guy orders a drink, third guy orders a drink. He comes to me. I have to start with a bowl of soup or an appetizer. The guys get used to my habits that differ somewhat from theirs.

But, no matter how much I would like to blend in and no matter how much I wish I could ease off my relatively strict regimen, I have to make it my priority to do whatever it takes to manage my diabetes well.

For me, the stakes are high. First of all, my livelihood depends on my physical health. Keep my body strong, I keep my job. Let my body slip below top condition, lose my job. It's that simple in my business. Second, I like to feel good. I don't like feeling tired all the time. I don't like to feel pressure build up behind my eyes. I don't like for my hands and feet to tingle and go numb. Third, I know that if I let up on managing my diabetes, not only will I lose my job and the advantage of feeling good, I'll be in danger of losing my eyesight, losing my kidneys, losing a foot to amputation. Ultimately, if I yield to the temptation of not managing my diabetes, I'll lose my life.

Is it hard to manage diabetes? Yes, it is. But these consequences are enough to get my attention. I want to live a long life. I want my body parts—my heart, my kidneys, my eyes—to work properly. I want my blood to keep circulating through my feet and fingers, so I'll still have them attached to my body in my old age.

So I do what I have to do. I'm thankful that I have been given so much to work with. My parents got me started right. They set me on a course to develop discipline and an inside toughness to tackle whatever life brings. If my father had been diagnosed with diabetes at my age, he wouldn't have whined about it. He would have gathered all his inner strength and, with God's help, he would have taken on diabetes and done his best to fight off its effects. I'm doing the same.

Through my youth, it never crossed my mind I would face a chronic disease. Few young people recognize how vulnerable they are to the destructive forces around them—accidents, injuries, diseases. I was certainly no exception. When I decided to attend the University of Iowa, I had no idea that the hospital would become as important a part of my world as the classroom and the football field.

\* \* \* \* \* \* \* \* \* \* \*

I had never felt better. Finishing up my junior year at the University of Iowa, I had nothing but confidence about the future. Ahead was a final collegiate season where I would be an offensive team captain and one of the senior leaders of a nationally ranked team. The adjustment to tight end from linebacker was complete; the upcoming year, with Coach Hayden Fry at the Hawkeye helm, held all the promise stored up in my boyhood dreams of college football.

Beyond the next year awaited the ultimate dream— a shot at the pros. It wouldn't be just a young boy's school yard fantasy anymore; this would be the real thing. . . the real draft, a real training camp, and, I hoped, the beginning of a long and productive professional football career.

The Iowa football team had been working out five times a week during the winter semester of 1984, preparing for the upcoming season. Thanks to concentrated training in the weight room, my 6-foot-5-inch frame had built to a solid 252 pounds, ample weight to drive a defensive end off the line of scrimmage or prevent a linebacker from reaching a ball carrier. Though I was strong enough to regularly bench press 315 pounds, the added bulk had not slowed me down. My time in the 40-yard dash had reached a new high of 4.6 seconds, nearly as fast as the running backs.

As the workouts progressed through March 1984, I felt I was reaching peak physical condition. At age 21, my body was coming into its own. I felt strong. I felt powerful. I felt confident. . . .

\* \* \* \* \* \* \*

"Jonathan, I think you may have diabetes."

It was as if I hadn't heard him at first. The team doctor, Dr. Johnson, was speaking to me in the examination room at the Student Health Clinic on April 11, 1984. But he had just used a word that did not register.

Diabetes?

"That's impossible," I thought.

"But, Doc, I've never been in better shape. I'm as strong as an ox. How could I have diabetes?"

"Well, I can't be certain. But I want you to go over to the diabetes clinic at the hospital and have some tests run."

Over the previous two or three weeks, I had felt progressively weaker. I lacked the stamina to push through my complete weightlifting routine, and I was struggling to bench press 275 pounds. My legs were weary after the first few minutes of drills on the practice field. My thirst was unquenchable, despite glass after glass of water. And I would need to urinate often, sometimes four or five times during the night.

In my senior year of high school, I had contracted mononucleosis and had to struggle through several weeks of recovery. This must be a relapse, I concluded. Though I had hoped the symptoms would clear up on their own, I finally decided to get checked out. I told Ed Crowley, the team trainer, at our afternoon workout one day that I thought I should see the team doctor.

After a urine test and an examination at the Student Health Clinic, the doctor quickly discounted the mononucleosis self-diagnosis I offered. He said my symptoms pointed to diabetes.

"It doesn't matter that you're in great shape, Jonathan," he explained, sympathetically but without softening the blow. "If your pancreas stops working. . . it stops working." He told me he would call over to the endocrine clinic at the University of Iowa Hospital and let them know I was coming.

"Hey, Doc," I said. "If that's what it is, will I still be able to play football?"

"Jonathan, this isn't going to end your life. If you manage it and control it properly, I don't see any reason why you won't be able to continue playing ball." Those words were a strand of hope in the net of despair closing in on me.

"Don't panic," he said. "I'm not even sure that you have diabetes. Just go to the clinic, and we'll know more." I shuffled out of his office, stunned.

Walking to the hospital, I had several minutes to sort through what the doctor had told me. The afternoon sun was shining brightly, giving a golden sheen to the campus buildings; the Iowa spring air was cool.

But an ominous cloud of dread hung over my head and blew through my thoughts. How could this happen to me? This kind of thing happens to other people, I thought, trying to grasp the implications of the doctor's words.

Just then, an eerie memory struck me. It was a spring day just like this some 20 years earlier that my grandmother on my mother's side had died. The clear sky and crisp air of that day in early spring had signaled the end of life on earth for my grandmother. Would this day see the death of my dreams? Of my strength? Of my health? I kept walking, but did not want to arrive.

I searched the doctor's words for whatever hope might be hidden in their meaning. Maybe he's wrong, I thought. After all, he's not a specialist. He said he wasn't sure. . . . I searched my memory for anything about diabetes, I thought back to a visit with my dad's family when I was about 9 years old. . . .

It seemed as though we had been driving all night to get to Muncie, Indiana, for this holiday visit with my dad's family. My dad, as was his habit when we embarked on a long trip, had roused us from our dreams about 4:00 in the morning. He loaded us into our big Dodge, four-door sedan and pulled onto the interstate. The back seat wasn't as comfortable as my bed had been, but I still curled up for a couple more hours of sleep.

When we arrived, my two brothers and I dashed to the door and thundered into my grandparents' house. Several other relatives, cousins, and aunts and uncles who lived in Muncie were also there; we greeted everyone and settled in for our week-long visit.

One afternoon, I was in the kitchen with Tony,

my 9-year-old cousin. He was unwrapping a needle and attaching it to a small tube with a clear solution in it. Quickly, painlessly, he thrust the point into his upper thigh and injected the solution.

At first, I looked away, thinking it would embarrass him if he knew I was watching.

"It's okay," he said, reassuring me. "It's just my medicine." He explained that he had diabetes. He had been diagnosed earlier that year and this procedure of injecting his own insulin shots was quite routine. That was the first time I remember hearing the word, "diabetes". . . .

As I neared the hospital, my mind searched the intervening 12 years since that visit for evidence of the effect of diabetes on my cousin. He seemed to be living a reasonably normal life, I thought. He played just as hard as we did. He looked healthy. How did he get the disease? Did he eat poorly? Not take care of himself?

My ignorance proved to be a breeding ground for anxiety. Frightening questions swarmed me like defensive linemen around a trapped quarterback. How could I have gotten a disease like this? Did I do something wrong? Why me?

What about football? Would I be able to play my senior season? Even if I could play, would any pro team draft me? Or would they see me as "handicapped"? How would I break the news to my teammates? Was I about to find out that today's workout was my last one with the team?

I had also held onto a boyhood dream of someday working in law enforcement like my dad. He spent most of his adult years working for the Parole Board in western Pennsylvania. Would any police force or law enforcement agency hire me if I had diabetes?

More immediate concerns haunted me as well.

What if they tell me I'm really sick and I can't even go to classes? Am I going to fall behind? Will I have to stay in the hospital? Will I be able to get to practice this afternoon, or will I have to come up with some explanation for Coach Fry?

I didn't have enough information to defend myself against this mental assault; all I could cling to were the doctor's assurances and my memories of my cousin who seemed to live a reasonably normal life despite his diabetes.

I held onto a glimmer of hope that the doctor was wrong. The tests at the clinic would be more extensive; perhaps their diagnosis would be different. If I could just hear those magic words: "There must have been some mistake. . . ."

## Initial Tests

The ten-minute walk seemed to take hours, but I arrived at the front door of the hospital. The receptionist at the endocrine clinic seemed to be expecting me. She invited me to sit down and said someone would be with me soon. After just a minute or two, an attractive nurse in her mid-30s stepped out and invited me to come back into the clinic. I wondered if my nervousness showed. She was relaxed.

"We don't see too many of the football players in here," she said jovially, as if this were just another routine day for her. "I've enjoyed watching you play." Her name was Linda Larson, and like most people on campus, she was an avid Hawkeye fan. With some effort, I managed a slight smile.

Linda explained that they would run some initial tests and that she would let me know later about the results. During the next hour, she fielded a steady barrage of my questions. Doing her best to ease my anxiety, she offered steady, straightforward answers.

The session turned out to be my first diabetes education class.

She explained that if I was developing diabetes, my pancreas was shutting down and slowing its production of insulin, which controls the level of sugar in my blood. During the initial "honeymoon period," when the disease is developing, symptoms begin but can be controlled with a combination of diet adjustments, exercise, and oral medication or insulin.

Though I left the clinic without knowing whether I had diabetes, I was breathing much easier. Even if I did have the disease, Linda had convinced me that it wouldn't mean the end of life as I had known it. She sent me out of the clinic back to my regular routine, so at least the experts were not pressing any panic buttons about my condition. I simply had to wait for the test results.

## Preliminary Diagnosis

Later that afternoon I was completing my weight routine at the football complex when the trainer came into the room.

"Hey, Jonathan, I need to see you in my office when you get finished." I assumed Ed had heard something. Slowly, deliberately, I finished up my workout, grabbed a towel and headed toward his office.

"Jonathan, the nurse from the clinic called. She said the tests indicate you are probably developing diabetes."

My expression didn't change.

"What does that mean?" I asked. "Do I have it or not?"

"That's all she said. She wants you to come in this week, and she'll fill you in on everything."

When I arrived for the appointment two days later, this time at the Hospital's Diabetes Clinic, Linda was waiting for me. She picked up where she had left off.

"Jonathan, the tests show that you are probably pre-diabetic and in the 'honeymoon period' of diabetes onset. That means that for now we will try to control your condition with oral medication along with a proper diet and exercise program."

I still didn't know exactly what all this meant, though she had begun the explanation on my first visit. Would I get worse? Might it go away? Would this medicine control my blood sugar for the rest of my life? And, as was always on my mind. . . .

"Will I still be able to play ball?"

"You're going to have to learn a new way to go through your daily life," she said. "But if you will eat properly and keep up your exercise routine, you should be able to continue a normal life."

"Including playing football?" I pressed her for specifics.

"Yes, including playing football." Once again, relief eased through me.

She continued her monologue about diet and exercise, adding that at some point my condition would have to be treated with insulin. But I began getting lost in the sea of information. And with the assurance that I could continue playing ball, and that medicine could help control the symptoms, my mind left the crisis mode and returned to more normal concerns.

"Chuck and Hap are probably waiting for me," I thought to myself, as she explained the role of the pancreas and the fluctuations of sugar levels in my bloodstream. I had arranged with two buddies from the football team, my roommate Hap Peterson, who played nose guard, and Chuck Long, our quarterback, to go out that day.

"It's very important that you follow the diet we're

going to set up for you," she said. I nodded, with a somewhat absent stare. Linda was just hitting full stride in her one-on-one training drill. But, satisfied that my condition did not represent the immediate tragedy I had feared, her list of cautions slipped past me as I waited for an opportunity to bring the conversation to a close.

## Parents' Visit

The remaining weeks of spring practice went well. The doctor at the diabetes clinic had confirmed my diagnosis; I did indeed have diabetes, but with the medicine he had prescribed, my strength returned, and the other symptoms I had complained of disappeared. I made a few of the diet adjustments Linda recommended: three solid meals a day, no late-night pizza, very little beer. I even intensified my workouts a bit, though my regular workout regimen was already demanding. She had given me a blood glucose monitor, so I periodically checked my blood sugar level.

Of course, my parents had been concerned when they learned of my diagnosis, but I worked hard at playing down its importance. They had a scheduled visit to campus coming up in just a few weeks for the annual Parents Day, and I assured them they would find me in good shape.

Once they arrived for the weekend, my mother started in right away with questions about my health.

"I'm fine," I kept assuring her. "There's nothing to worry about."

"Well, what did the doctors tell you," she quizzed. "How long will this medicine be effective?"

She drilled me with a stream of questions, more questions than even I had asked. Then she started in on a campaign to see the doctor. She was determined, but I resisted strongly. I didn't want her to escalate this into a medical emergency. I wanted her to leave the matter for me to handle.

The highlight of the Parents Day weekend was the spring game, followed by a picnic for the athletes' families to meet the team and the coaches. She never got to the doctor that weekend, but she did run into Ed, our trainer, at the picnic. He seemed to satisfy her with the reassurance that I was doing fine.

## Parental Concern

My mother's concern was no surprise. My parents have always cared deeply about my two older brothers and me and have always been intensely involved in our lives. Throughout high school, my mother was not only in the stands for every game, but she was also volunteering to cook meals for the team, helping organize fund-raising events, and doing whatever she could behind the scenes to support our involvement in sports and other activities. Meanwhile, she was also working full time; she taught second grade in the public schools in the Pittsburgh area for 34 years.

To this day when I go home, she'll be on me about taking care of myself. "Jonathan, where's your coat?" she'll say if I head toward the door on a chilly day. "Mom, I'm a full-grown adult. Don't you think I'm old enough to figure out whether to wear a coat or not?" I'll say with a smile. I guess I still enjoy the attention.

My father was also tuned in to our lives while we were growing up. If we did something wrong, he'd be the first to be on us. But if someone did us wrong, he would be in that person's face the next day, asking for an explanation.

One day when I was in high school, I was playing basketball in the school gym with some friends. A guy passed me a ball, but I had to move to my left to get it. In the flurry of activity on the court, I scrambled to the ball and jerked it toward my chest to keep the opponent from getting it. I felt a little contact but thought nothing of it. With 10 big guys scrambling around on the court in an aggressive game of basketball, most contact goes unnoticed. It turned out that I had accidentally bumped one of the gym teachers, who had been walking along the side of the court. He was a relatively small man, and the impact knocked him to the floor.

He jumped up and started shouting, moving toward me. We stopped the game. My buddies were all looking on, wondering what he was so upset about.

"I'm sorry," I said immediately. "I didn't see you there."

My explanation did not matter; he was convinced I had knocked him down on purpose.

"Just because you're an athlete, you think you own the building, and you don't have to respect anyone else," he screamed.

Then, with the rage reddening his face, he charged toward me. I don't know what he thought he was going to do. He was just a small guy, and even by this time in high school I had reached about 6 feet, 4 inches and 205 pounds. My friends got between us. It takes a lot to push me to the point of losing my temper, but he had brought me right to the edge. He was out of control.

We ended up in the principal's office. The principal, a reasonable man, listened to the story, then called me aside into a separate office. This gym teacher has a problem, he explained, asking me to forget about the incident. There's no need to get your father involved, he added, knowing from past encounters that my father would take this matter seriously and that the school could face severe consequences from a teacher assaulting a student. I promised to keep quiet.

But so many people had witnessed the event that

word got back to my father. He asked me about it, and I tried to brush it off as a brief argument.

"It was no big deal," I said.

He wasn't satisfied. He announced he would be in the principal's office first thing Monday morning to get to the bottom of this. When we went in that Monday, my dad and I sat down with the principal and the coach. The principal had also asked one of my football coaches to stand by in case things got out of hand. I knew the principal had not wanted to deal with my dad. My father was certainly not prone to violence. But there could be times when in his mind events would justify strong action. A teacher, an individual in a position of responsibility with young people, losing control and assaulting one of his boys might qualify as one of those times.

After reviewing the events, my dad asked me to leave the room. He did not repeat to me what he told the teacher.

Later I asked the other football coach what happened. He said my dad put his finger in that man's face, asking if he had come at his son. At first, the little coach denied it, but finally he conceded that he had. My dad warned him, quite vehemently, never to lay a hand on his son—or that teacher would have to deal with him. And he wouldn't be so peaceful the next time. I think my dad made his point.

As well as paying close attention to my brothers' and my lives, he was also involved with people in the community, helping in whatever ways he could. He would take a guy in the neighborhood to the doctor, or give an elderly person a ride up the hill.

My leaving home for college didn't disrupt my parents' involvement in my life. Often, my parents would drive all night from Pittsburgh to Iowa City to come to a Hawkeye game. In fact, during my senior season they came to every conference game. They are, by far, my number one fans.

So, I was not surprised by my mother's aggressive interest in my medical condition during their visit to the Iowa campus in that spring of 1984. The fact that I was nearly through with college and 800 miles from home had done nothing to dampen her maternal instincts. I also knew that for every question she asked aloud, my father was asking the same thing to himself. They cared, and I appreciated it. I did not, however, want them to create a crisis. As far as I was concerned, my condition was under control.

# CHAPTER
## 2

# DOCTOR
# OF
# MY OWN BODY

"**M**an, those jeans are falling off you," Hap Peterson said as I was leaving our dormitory room for a class one day in late October 1984, during the fall semester of my senior year. "Are you losing weight?"

"No," I replied quickly. "I bought these last spring when I had bulked up a lot. They're just too big for me."

It was a lie. I had bought the jeans near the beginning of that semester when I weighed my normal 230 pounds. Now, a couple of months into the semester and eight games into the football season, my weight was down to 220.

Through the summer I had stayed in Iowa City, working a couple of jobs and keeping up with my regular workout routine to prepare for this season. The oral medication, along with my regular exercise routine and somewhat improved dietary habits, was still controlling my blood sugar levels adequately.

I had remained strong through the preseason workouts and the first several games of the season. Coach Snyder, our offensive coordinator, had worked me into the heart of the offensive scheme. Since I would be one of the senior team leaders, he thought it would be important for me to be an integral part of the offense.

As a result, Chuck Long was throwing me my fair share of passes, and I was building up some good senior season statistics, especially for a tight end. Every time we took the field, I was contributing.

By mid-October, after our first several games, I began to notice once again that I was having to urinate more often than normal during the day and several times at night. My body was slower bouncing back after workouts and games. I was feeling more and more sluggish, and when I would check my blood sugar level, it would be high much more frequently than it had been.

Hap wasn't the only one who noticed my weight loss. Several people commented that I looked thinner. Every player tends to lose some weight from the wear and tear of a football season, so I was able to brush off the questions by claiming mine to be normal mid-season weight loss.

Each inquiry drove me deeper into hiding. Privately, I knew that my pancreas was shutting down. Linda Larson had warned me that I would begin experiencing these kinds of symptoms at some point as my "honeymoon period" reached its end. I knew my insulin-free days were about over. But rather than reporting into the clinic and keeping the medical staff informed about my condition, I stubbornly resolved to handle the situation myself.

When I considered my dilemma, I saw a team that had a legitimate shot at a conference championship and the Rose Bowl, the hope of any Big Ten college football player. As a team captain, I felt I had a role to play to help get us there. We had key games coming up in November that would determine the conference championship. Then the final plum of the schedule was a non-conference game December 1 in Hawaii, one road trip I did not want to miss. Besides, I was having my best season ever, accumulating some impressive pass-catching statistics. I wanted nothing to disrupt this season—including diabetes.

Rather than yield to the conclusion my symptoms were announcing—namely, that my body needed insulin—I determined to keep pushing through the season. I even doubled my dosage of medicine, slipping in an extra pill in hopes of bringing my sugar level down. I scrutinized my diet more closely than ever and made sure to keep up my exercise routine, even though I didn't feel up to it. I even tried to add a few repetitions on the weights, again trying to bring the sugar level down. But the readings on my glucose monitor told me that my condition was worsening.

Despite all this, though, my performance on the field did not suffer. Through the end of October and the beginning of November, I kept playing every game, keeping quiet about my symptoms.

## Road to the Rose Bowl

With our conference record at 5-2-1, we faced a pivotal game November 10 with Michigan State. The previous week we had lost a couple of key players in a game against Wisconsin that had ended in a disappointing tie. Chuck had banged up his knee, so he was not at full strength. Ronnie Harmon, one of our running backs, had broken his leg and was gone for the season. But we had beaten Michigan State several years in a row, and we were determined to take them again.

It was a warm day for November, about 65 degrees. We had fought hard to take this game despite missing some key players, but we were down by a touchdown in the fourth quarter. We marched down the field on a final drive and reached the four-yard line. On a third down play, Chuck, who had come in to play the second half, called a pass play. From my tight end spot, I took off on a route into the end zone and worked free of the defensive back. Chuck fired a pass right into my belly—TOUCHDOWN! That brought the score to 17-16.

Rather than settling for a tie, which would have been our second in as many weeks, Coach Fry decided to go for a two point conversion—all or nothing. We tried a quarterback option. Chuck took the snap and ran down the line of scrimmage. He saw an opening and turned up field, charging toward the end zone. The linebacker stepped up and made contact, bringing Chuck down inches from the goal line.

We tried an onside kick but a Michigan State player fell on the ball. Final score, 17-16—a heartbreaking loss.

All of us had poured every ounce of strength out on that field, scratching and clawing to win that game, and everyone was dragging when it was over. So it did not seem out of the ordinary for me to sit slumped on the stool by my locker, completely drained of energy. Ed came by, as he did after every game, and asked how I was doing, mainly checking for scrapes and bruises that might need attention.

"Fine," I said, being careful not to give any indication that I was struggling more than usual. He moved on to the next player.

But by Monday, the other guys had bounced back and were ready to go at it again on the practice field and in the weight room. But I was still dragging Monday, Tuesday, and Wednesday, having to force myself through the workouts. My body just wasn't responding.

Ed noticed I was struggling through my workouts and that my weight was down. He was concerned and suggested that I bring in the chart I used to record my blood sugar levels. During those weeks, I had made sure that I only recorded the readings I took before meals or after workouts, when my levels would tend to be lower. As I had hoped, the chart satisfied him. Like me, the training staff was new to diabetes, and it didn't occur to Ed to ask when I had taken the readings.

Our final conference game was November 17 in Minneapolis against the University of Minnesota. This would be the day we would find out which Big Ten team would head for Pasadena, Calif., to face the Pac-10 conference champion in the Rose Bowl. We were confident we could beat Minnesota. But if Ohio State beat Michigan in their matchup that afternoon, the Buckeyes would be the Big-10 champions, and we would be watching the Rose Bowl on television.

Several guys gathered in one of our Minneapolis hotel rooms to watch the first half of the Ohio State-Michigan game. It was still close when we left for the Humphreydome. But during our pregame workout, we heard the announcement over the loudspeaker: Ohio State had defeated Michigan. This was the Buckeyes' year.

Heads were lowered all over our side of the field. Coach Fry gathered us in the locker room and delivered one of his patented speeches aimed at stirring us to play for pride. But we just couldn't shake the Ohio State news. They were tasting what we had hungered for the entire season. We ended up just going through the motions and let that game slip through our fingers. We felt our season had slipped away as well.

Once again, after the game, Ed stopped by.

"How are you doing, Jonathan?"

"Fine," I said, as usual, but I was getting worse. I didn't know how much longer I could go on. My body barely had enough energy to get my uniform and pads off and get to the shower.

We had a week off for Thanksgiving before leaving for Hawaii for our final regular season game. I flew home to Pittsburgh to spend the holiday with my parents. Throughout the long weekend, I was careful not to give them any indication about my condition, though I didn't feel up to doing anything but lie on the couch. I felt worse than ever; my primary activity was trips to the bathroom to urinate. With my weight now down to around 210, my energy level had not bounced back even after nearly a week of rest following the Minnesota game.

"I'm going to have to fatten you up, Jonathan," my mother said, noticing my weight loss of 35 pounds since the summer. "You're wasting away."

I just chuckled, then turned away to hide my slight grimace.

When the team had dispersed for Thanksgiving, we had not expected to be playing in a bowl game that year. But while I was at my parents' home, Coach Fry called and said he had received a bid invitation from the Freedom Bowl officials. Since I was one of the captains, he wanted to get my reaction.

"Should we go?" he asked.

"Heck yes," I said without hesitating, again ignoring my own deteriorating condition. Iowa had been to a bowl game for several years in a row. I certainly didn't want to be a captain of the team that broke the string. This would be a chance for the players to conclude the season on a more positive note.

After hanging up I wondered how long I could keep going. Could I make it through the Hawaii trip? Could I make it until after Christmas for the Freedom Bowl?

By this time, I was starting to feel tingling sensations in my fingers and toes. My eyes had begun to hurt. I had lost so much weight I could barely keep my pants on. My sugar levels were regularly beyond the normal zone. I was getting scared.

But I still couldn't bear the thought of cutting

short my senior season. If I reported my symptoms and sugar level readings to the doctor now, he would likely keep me from going to Hawaii. No way, I thought. Thoughts of that Hawaii beach had tantalized me all year; the trip represented a reward to the players after a long, hard season.

"After the Hawaii game," I thought. "After the Hawaii game, I've got to tell somebody." Even though it might mean missing the Freedom Bowl, I decided that the next game was as far as I could go.

## Aloha

As soon as we returned to campus after Thanksgiving, the team packed up and flew off to Hawaii. Coach Fry gave us a couple of days to relax and enjoy the Pacific sun before starting in on our workout schedule. On one hand it was a relief to not have to gather up the strength for a hard workout. On the other hand it was those strenuous workouts that helped drive down my blood sugar level. But I was feeling well enough to enjoy a surfboard and catamaran, swim in the ocean, and shop for souvenirs. We stayed at a gorgeous hotel with an inside waterfall—right on the beach. I was extremely careful about what I ate, concentrating on the fresh fruits and light foods. Even when we started practicing later in the week, the workouts would only last for about an hour and a half. They didn't interfere with the relaxation, but neither did they help much with my sugar level. Fortunately for me, the December temperatures were in the 80s, so I could at least break a good sweat with a little exertion.

Once game day came, I began to feel a sense of relief. The week under the Pacific sun had been enjoyable; now I was ready to play the game and perhaps let my season—along with my insulin-free life—come to a close. Oddly enough, considering the stress my body was experiencing, I had my best game of the season: seven catches, 77 yards, and a touchdown—a good closing chapter to the regular season of my senior year at Iowa.

After the game, I sat on a stool in the locker room, waiting for Ed to make his rounds.

"You all right?" he said.

"Yeah, I'm all right," I said, leaning over to cut the tape off my ankles. "But I think my sugars have gotten way out of control. When we get back, I think we need to call Linda and get me over to the clinic."

He stepped closer to me. "How long have you known this?"

"The last month or so. . . . I've been going kind of haywire," I said. "But I didn't want to tell you till after the game."

"Are you crazy?" he said, angrily. "You kept this from me all this time?"

"Well, I'm sorry," I said, like a criminal confessing to the local sheriff.

Finally, my private anguish had broken through the surface. Someone else knew. Even though he was upset that I had not let him know before, I was relieved that Ed had entered my private world. Now I would get the help I knew I needed. No longer would I have to convince the people around me that everything was fine. It wasn't.

## Hospital Stay

After returning from Hawaii, Ed contacted the Diabetes Clinic and set up an appointment for me on Thursday, December 6. This time, I was eager to get to the clinic. Rather than wrestling with fears about the future, I was breathing easier as I neared the front door, knowing help was waiting. I have always been a person who tries to handle problems on my own, sometimes more stubbornly than I should. But this was a battle I wasn't going to win alone. Hiding for weeks in my silence and half-truths had wearied me. I didn't want to feel sick anymore. Pulling open the clinic door, I walked into a new chapter in my life.

I told the doctor my blood sugar levels had been ranging from 250 to 350 recently, and I explained my other symptoms. He concluded that the oral medications were no longer doing the job; he wanted me in the hospital right away to begin insulin therapy.

When I showed up at the hospital the next morning, an aide came and showed me to a room. An initial blood test showed my sugar level at 454. In less than an hour, a nurse was at my bedside, mixing clear fluids together in a syringe. My honeymoon period was clearly over; my pancreas was no longer secreting enough insulin into my system. Unless the researchers find a cure for diabetes, I will need insulin injections for the rest of my life.

"Do you want me to give you the first shot? Or do you want to do it yourself?" she said, matter-of-factly.

"I'll do it," I said, falling back on my instincts to take care of myself. She must have discerned the hesitation in my voice. As much as I'm able to knock heads on the football field with 280-pound defensive linemen, that tiny, sharp needle intimidated me.

"Let me just show you the first time," she said.

The nurse explained the procedure as she prepared the shot. She showed me how to mix the two different types of insulin the doctor had prescribed for me and how to check for air bubbles in the syringe. Then she explained that the shot needed to go into the fatty tissue, not a vein, so that it could move through my body.

After she left, I lay back in the bed and, for the first time in several weeks, relaxed. I knew I was in the right place. Everything else, like football and classes, would have to be on hold for awhile. The only item on my agenda at that point was getting my sugar level down and stabilized.

Linda stopped by later that day. Her presence was reassuring. Only a few people were aware of the changes I would be facing. She was one who understood. As a friend as well as a nurse, she tried again to educate me. This time I was a far more attentive student. I don't like feeling sick, and I knew I would have to learn about managing this disease to avoid the kind of experience I had been through over the last several weeks.

Once again, Linda instructed me about how insulin helps my body process sugar, about food groups, about the effects of exercise. She explained that my sugar level needed to stay within the range of 80 to 150 or so. In my case, she said, because I work out so hard, it would not be a problem if my sugar level reached as high as 180 before a workout. The exertion and sweating would bring it down to an appropriate level. She suggested always having a snack or special tablets with me in case my blood sugar were to drop too low, so I could quickly get some sugar into my system. She told me all about food exchanges and how to balance my diet, about proteins and carbohydrates. I could go out to eat as often as I wanted to, she said, but I would have to ask about the ingredients in certain foods. I had to know what was entering my body, so I could anticipate the effect that food would have.

Giving shots would become second nature, she assured me, though it would be awkward at first. I would need to move the shots around so that one area did not develop fatty deposits or get too sore. She suggested starting in my upper thighs. One shot a day to start with, she said.

"That's a lot to learn at one time, isn't it?" she said.

"Yeah, I don't know if I'm going to remember all that," I said, shaking my head.

"You'll catch on," she said. "The main point is that you are the one who must take charge of your own body."

My motivation picked up when she listed some of the complications that can result from not taking care of diabetes properly. Like amputation of feet from loss of circulation. Like blindness. But, to be honest, though it is a little embarrassing, she mentioned one side effect that startled me even more than the others: impotence. No thank you.

I had always valued a healthy body, a strong physique, and I had been willing to pay the price to maintain it. Now the cost was going up. Now the cost included extra care about diet, extra attention during exercise, insulin shots, frequent finger pricks to check my sugar level. I would have to become the doctor of my own body, learning about its processes and fine-tuning my own lifestyle to accommodate it. These days in the hospital were the beginning of my personal medical school training, with Linda serving as my primary instructor.

Though I was ready to dive into these medical studies, learn about the disease and how to control it, I still had that one predominant question about the future:

"Linda, what about football? Will I still be able to play?"

She smiled, amused at my persistence.

"You know who Jackie Robinson is, don't you?" she asked, as we were discussing the impact my condition would have on the rest of my life.

"Sure."

"Did you know he had diabetes?" she asked, trying

to prove that diabetes did not have to rob me of what I could accomplish. She just about had me convinced.

## Party Time

Over the next couple of days, the doctors and nurses watched my sugar levels continually. My levels seemed to be staying stubbornly up over 250, so they kept adjusting my insulin and waiting to see some changes in the numbers.

During those first days in the hospital, I had no phone calls or visitors—except for Hap, my friend Nick, and the trainers, who were the only ones who knew I was there. I had asked them not to tell anyone I was in the hospital. Hap had asked if I wanted him to call my parents, but I didn't even want them to know until my condition was more under control.

I was glad to be getting the medical attention I needed. In the hospital environment the doctors and nurses were attuned to the physical and emotional adjustments a person beginning insulin therapy had to make. But I wasn't sure what it would be like out of the hospital with my friends, my teammates, my coaches, my family. How would they respond to me?

What I dreaded most was that people might feel sorry for me and feel as if they had to treat me with kid gloves. Yes, I had gotten sick. Yes, my blood sugar levels had soared out of control. Yes, I was in the hospital with a serious medical condition. And yes, my body would now need insulin because my pancreas was not functioning. But those facts did not add up to my wanting sympathy.

On Saturday, the second day of my hospital stay, my friend Nick and his girlfriend had planned a party. Nick came by to see me and encouraged me to ask Linda if I could come. It would be a season-ending get-together with several of my teammates along with a few other friends. I was a little apprehensive about how people might react to me if they knew I had been in the hospital because of my diabetes, but I wanted to go. I had certainly seen enough of the walls of my hospital room. Linda warned me not to eat or drink anything, but she didn't object to my slipping out for a couple of hours.

Once I arrived at the party, I couldn't tell whether my friends were reacting differently to me. "How many of these people know where I've been," I wondered, scanning the familiar faces. "And if they know I've been in the hospital, do they know why?" Hap and Nick knew. Nick probably had told his girlfriend. I spoke with several people through the evening, but it was difficult to relax with them. Were they wondering about my condition? Did they want to ask if something was wrong but didn't want to be rude? It was awkward. I was especially afraid that some self-appointed comic would have found out I was in the hospital and would pop up in the crowd and try for a few laughs at my expense. Fortunately, nothing like that happened. After a couple of hours, Nick took me back to my hospital room.

## Return to the Weight Room

On Monday, after four days in the hospital, I suggested that maybe a good workout would help drive my sugar level down. After all, Linda had spoken about the importance of exercise. Years before, doctors had discouraged people with diabetes from trying intensive workouts but now the general wisdom was that it could be helpful. I would just have to pay close attention to my body's responses.

"How can I learn if you won't let me do anything?" I argued to Linda, desperate for some kind of physical activity. After talking with the doctor, Linda gave the go-ahead, knowing that I needed to learn what the fluctuations in my blood sugar would feel like now that I was on insulin. She went over the sensations I would experience if my blood sugar level got too low.

"Get a good workout. Get a good sweat going," she said. "But don't overdo it." Her emphasis was on the final phrase.

I checked in with Ed, and he and a student trainer stood by as I started my regular workout. I planned to go through each exercise, reducing my normal repetitions. We had also notified the strength coach, Coach Dervich, that I was trying a full workout. Periodically, he asked a little nervously how I was doing. Each time I told him I felt good. Beads of sweat had popped out on my forehead, and patches of dampness were showing up on my gray shirt. I was like a fish happy to be back in water. I was back in the football weight room where I had spent so much time during my college years.

After my full routine, I stood up, dripping sweat, and looked over toward Ed, ready to report on a successful workout. But just then, I started feeling a little strange. My arms started to quiver; then my legs began quivering too. Shortly I was quaking all over, and my heart was racing in high gear.

"Ed," I said, trying to keep calm. "I think I went too low."

Ed sprang to my side and helped me over to a bench. "Go get him a soda—now!" he shouted to the student trainer. Coach Dervich, who had remained nearby in the training room, was at my side in seconds. The student trainer fumbled with his quarters at the machine, then raced back toward me with a Mountain Dew in hand. I gulped it down. The shaking continued. My heart was still pounding.

"Get him another one," Ed shouted, this time tossing him the key to the machine. Ed's eyes were sharply focused, fixed on my face. He was ready to grab the phone and get a hospital emergency crew there immediately.

The second soda started to make a difference, lifting my sugar level toward the normal range. The shaking slowed, then ultimately stopped; my heart rate settled back to normal. The student brought me a third soda, and I poured down about half of that. I sat still for about 25 minutes, a little shaken by the incident, but feeling much better. Ed sat with me, making sure I was stable, then sent the student trainer to walk with me back to the hospital.

"How did it go?" Linda asked when I got back to my room.

"There was a little problem," I said, having recovered enough to show a slight grin.

"What happened?" she said.

"Maybe I pushed a little too hard. I was feeling good, so I figured I could do a few more reps than I planned on," I said. "Then it was like a truck hit me."

"What did you do?"

"Grabbed a couple of sodas, three actually."

She said that now I'd had a good lesson in diabetes management, taken a new step in being the doctor of my own body. Now I would know what it felt like when my blood sugar got low.

"Next time it won't be so alarming," she said. "You'll know what to do."

She indicated that we had overreacted a bit, chuckling briefly as she checked my blood sugar level on her monitor. Those two and a half sodas had pushed my sugar level back up too high. One 12-ounce can probably would have been sufficient, she said.

I shook my head back and forth slowly.

"This is complicated," I said.

The next day, after five days in the hospital, I

agreed with the doctor that I was ready to go. He was satisfied that my blood sugar level had stabilized and the insulin dosage was appropriate. So they loaded me up with needles and syringes, a prescription for insulin, and a card to remind me of an appointment at the clinic two days later.

## All-America Tight End

The football awards banquet was scheduled for the next weekend. When the awards presentation began, Coach Fry announced that I had been honored as a first team All-America tight end by the Gannett News agency, second team All Big Ten by United Press International, and honorable mention All Big Ten by the Associated Press. I accepted the awards, then thanked Coach Fry, the rest of the coaching staff, and my teammates for their help in my success. I thanked Coach Snyder, the offensive coordinator, for adjusting the offensive scheme to get the tight end much more involved in the offense. That was the most significant factor leading to my senior season statistics of 42 catches, 512 yards, for 6 touchdowns. I thanked Coach Alvarez for recruiting me; he had become not only a coach but a friend. He often spoke to my dad on the phone and kept him up to date on my progress at Iowa.

Afterward, Hap's father shook my hand and asked how I was feeling. Hap had told him that I had been diagnosed with diabetes and that I had been in the hospital. The Petersons had become like second parents to me, and I appreciated their concern. I assured them I was doing much better now. Ironically, years later, Hap's dad would develop diabetes as well.

"Jonathan, do you want to join us to get something to eat?" Hap's dad asked, after the last award was given.

"No, thanks," I said. "I'm just going to head back

to my room and relax. . . . I've got something I have to do."

Back in my room, I picked up the phone and dialed the area code for western Pennsylvania, then my parents' number. My mom answered. I had decided to wait to call them until the alarming part of my ordeal was over. I knew how they would react, and I didn't want to add another worry to their lives.

"I'm coming out tomorrow!" my mom said as soon as I gave her my news.

"No, Mom, it's not necessary. You don't need to come out."

"Look, son, I'm coming out tomorrow. I'll check the flights and be there as early as possible."

She was responding just as I had predicted.

"Mom, I'm fine. Everything's under control."

"You always say you're fine," she snapped back. "If you're so fine, how come you've been in the hospital for a week!"

"Mom, it's really under control. I've been in the hospital, but I'm learning what I have to do to take care of this. It's no big deal."

Finally, she calmed down; I had convinced her that it was not an emergency. I assured her that I would ask Linda to call her to explain all the details. That seemed to satisfy her. We agreed to stick with the plan of meeting later that month in Anaheim for the Freedom Bowl game. We would have a chance to go over everything then.

# CHAPTER
### 3

## DRAFT DAY

"**H**ello."

"Good morning, may I speak to Jonathan Hayes, please?"

"This is he."

"Jonathan, this is Dave Kendall of the Kansas City Chiefs. . . ."

The National Football League draft had begun early Tuesday morning, April 30, 1985. Teams had 30 minutes each in the first round to pick their player, so by around 11:00 a.m. I knew that several teams had made their selections. I was not sure exactly where the Chiefs fell in the order—the middle of the pack somewhere, I thought.

"We wanted to check on how you are doing health-wise," he continued. Dave Kendall was the trainer for the Chiefs.

"I'm doing fine," I said, without elaboration.

### Freedom Bowl

After I had left the hospital four months earlier, we had one more game to play that season—the Freedom Bowl, scheduled for Dec. 26. Of course I had been prepared for the possibility that I might have to miss it. After my hospital stay, though, the doctor had given me the go-ahead to return to practice and, if I felt up to it, to prepare for the game.

The practices over those two weeks in December 1984 had served as my personal experiment as a football player with insulin-dependent diabetes. I worked hard during the practices, paying attention to how I felt, learning more about how my body would react to physical exertion. The Gatorade was always handy for the times I felt as if my blood sugar might be dropping. I experimented with different eating patterns, adding a little more to my meals before and after practices, taking snacks periodically, trying to find the best way to keep my blood sugar within the appropriate levels.

Meanwhile, the doctors were also still adjusting my insulin dosage, watching my body's reactions and searching for the proper level for my particular body type and relatively heavy workout regimen.

When we flew to Anaheim, Calif., right after Christmas, the Freedom Bowl game would be my first chance to find out how I could perform under game conditions. Though this bowl game lacked some of the glamour of the more prestigious New Year's Day games, we were glad, especially those of us who were seniors, for the chance to make our final statement about the quality of the 1984 Iowa Hawkeye football team.

The Texas Longhorns had come into Anaheim making predictions of their dominance and commenting about the "big, slow farm boys from Iowa." We quietly agreed we would make them eat every word they uttered and take back every cocky glance they shot toward us during the pre-game events.

Suffice it to say that after the game, their Longhorn lips were sealed. We pummeled them and left them whimpering off the field from a 55-17 drubbing. Chuck had thrown the first and last touchdown passes to me, one in the first quarter and another in the third quarter. By the fourth quarter, most of the regulars were on the sideline, cheering on the younger back-up players. At the end of the game, I had three catches for 70 yards and two touchdowns, my most productive game of the season.

I had approached the game with apprehension: Can I still play well? My weight was headed back up toward normal by this time, but would my strength be there? Would my quickness remain? Would my mind be tough enough to compete? The team's win and my individual statistics pleased me, but that game answered all my internal questions. I performed as well as I had in any game. I could still play football.

So, when the questions came on draft day regarding my diabetes, I could answer in good conscience that I would be able to report to training camp in excellent health.

"Do you have your diabetes under control?" Dave Kendall asked.

"Yeah, I do. I'm not having any problems at all."

I had been through a round of physicals since the season ended. Doctors from the New York Jets, the Seattle Seahawks, and the Chiefs had looked me over. Each time, I waited to see how much they would investigate my diabetes. I never tried to cover it up, although I never volunteered any information beyond what was necessary.

Remarkably, none of the doctors seemed overly concerned. They seemed more intent on checking my knees and joints than my blood sugar levels. When they did inquire, I simply told them my diabetes was under control and that I had continued playing with no problems last year. I encouraged them to contact my doctor in Iowa City and the Hawkeyes' trainer if they wanted to know more. Their seeming indifference to such a serious disease surprised me—but it was a great relief. It almost seemed like they viewed diabetes like a bad cold or a case of the flu.

When I assured Dave Kendall that I had my diabetes under control, he seemed satisfied and said he was simply doing some routine preliminary checks to brief the Chiefs' officials as they prepared for their 1985 draft selections.

My roommates huddled around me during the brief conversation, waiting expectantly to find out if that was "the call." I told them it was just a preliminary contact from the Chiefs.

## Party Preparations

That morning I had slept in, but I awakened to strange noises that I quickly recognized as party preparations. Doors were slamming, the vacuum cleaner was running, Hap and Mike Haight were scurrying around picking up trash, dusting off table tops, washing dishes. This was indeed a strange scene; usually it was only Mike and me who kept the place from being mistaken for an illegal trash dump. They had rolled in a couple of kegs of beer and were clearly poised for celebration.

"Oh no," I thought to myself, cringing as I got up and saw the enthusiasm on their faces. I wanted a quiet day—time alone or perhaps with just a few friends.

Yes, I was excited. Yet I knew there were no guarantees on draft day. Sharing joy with a crowd is one thing, but what do you do with disappointment? I would rather deal with that alone. I knew the stories of a player getting cocky on draft day, only to face embarrassment as the rounds proceeded and the phone remained silent.

To my great relief, I found out that no one would be showing up till later in the day. The morning would be reasonably quiet. I ate breakfast, took my medicine, and settled in for a John Wayne movie. Hap had rented several of my favorites to help me relax.

The draft was televised, but we did not have cable TV in our apartment. I couldn't go elsewhere to watch because I had to stay by my phone. Besides, it would be far too agonizing to listen to every name called, waiting to hear if the next one might be mine. Chuck, who had chosen to play at Iowa for one more year, and Nick were each a few blocks away at their girlfriends' apartments watching on ESPN. Every so often one of them would drop over to update us on the proceedings.

About twenty minutes after the conversation with Dave Kendall, the phone rang again. I still thought it was too early for a team to call—at that time of day it would still be early first round.

"Hello, Jonathan, we just wanted to make sure that you are eligible for the draft," said the voice on the other end. The man identified himself as a representative of the New York Giants.

"Yes, I am," I told him. That's all he wanted to know, so the quiet vigil continued. Now, though, with the Giants inquiring about my eligibility, possibilities began to swirl in my mind.

## Draft Decisions

It had been rumored that the Giants were looking for a tight end in the draft and that they might be interested in me. In my conversations with agents and the coaching staff, I had also heard reports that the Chicago Bears might draft a tight end early. They had been pleased, I was told, with the way other Iowa players had performed at the professional level. We ran a relatively complex offense at Iowa, so the adjustment to the pro offenses was not so overwhelming for our guys.

Although the speculations of scouts and agents are nothing to rely on, the talk on the street had been that I would likely be a first or second round pick, probably the third player from Iowa taken. Word was that Owen Gill, a running back, and George Little, a defensive lineman, would be taken ahead of me.

The decision to enter the draft had not been easy. Though Chuck and I had been at Iowa four years, we had the option of staying for a fifth year of eligibility because of an NCAA rule change. Many evenings during the first several weeks of the winter semester of 1985 Chuck and I would sit at the kitchen table in the apartment we had moved into and talk about the factors to consider. We really had become close friends, and another year at Iowa with the quarterback-tight end tandem in place could have been an awesome experience with the high-powered offense we had. Especially since we hadn't reached our goal of the conference championship and the Rose Bowl that senior year, we speculated about what one more year together might bring. Ultimately, I knew that my decision would have to extend beyond college-life sentiments and that Chuck and I would each have to make our own choices.

Coach Fry tried to persuade me to stay at Iowa another year. The scouts, he told me, were saying I had pro potential at tight end but that I still needed to develop since I had only moved to the position from linebacker the year before. According to him, the scouts were predicting the middle rounds if I entered the draft. Anytime I gave the impression in our discussions that I might consider leaving Iowa, he would take over the conversation and insist that I take plenty of time to think about it, not to rush into a decision.

My dad spoke with me often about the decision. His primary concern was simply that I complete my degree, but he knew that I could finish the few hours I had remaining even if I began a professional career. He encouraged me to make a list of the positives and negatives associated with the decision, then make my best call. Neither choice would be wrong, he assured me, adding that he would support me either way. At this stage of my life, my dad thought it was important for this decision to be fully mine.

Finally, after several weeks of agonizing, Chuck made his decision. He would stay for another year at the University of Iowa. His news delighted Hawkeye fans everywhere, and most fans and reporters expected me to follow suit. A few days later, though, I made my decision public: I would enter the National Football League draft.

"I'm going to take my shot," I told Coach Fry one day in his office in February.

His look soured. "I think you're making a bad decision," he said slowly, after several moments of silence. He had expected his perspective to prevail and influence my choice.

"I respect you for your opinion and your help and all you've done for me," I told him, "but I'm going to take my shot at the draft."

This was my time to seize the opportunity for a professional career, I had concluded. While another year at Iowa might have become a tremendous culmination of my college experience and perhaps even increased my value in the eyes of a pro team, that option offered no guarantees either. Maybe we could rewrite the college record books. On the other hand, an injury could eliminate my chance at the pro dream.

Even if a professional football career did not work out, I was ready to face the future with my college football days behind me. Pro ball or not, it was time to move on.

It had all seemed clear back in February, but as the morning of draft day progressed, I thought back on Coach Fry's advice. Had I made a mistake? Would the first several rounds go by without my name being entered as a draft choice? Might I have been a first or second round selection if I had waited one more year? Would I look back on my decision as the most foolish thing I had ever done? I started getting edgier, wondering how far the draft had proceeded. They were probably in the second round by this time, I calculated.

The phone rang again. Instinctively, I sprang toward the receiver but stopped myself. Letting it ring again, I gathered my composure and lifted the receiver slowly to my ear.

"Hello," I said, waiting to hear which team was on the line.

"Hi, Jonathan, it's me. . . . Just wanted to check on how you're holding up. . . ."

"Dad, get off the phone!" I said. I couldn't believe my father was tying up the line. As respectfully as I could, but quite abruptly, I promised I would call him as soon as I got "the call."

That would be just great, I thought, if someone had tried to call and heard a busy signal—I would be the last to know I was drafted!

The feeling nagged me that something was going to go wrong, that some little hitch would interfere with my being drafted. Two days before, when I assumed everything was in order, the Iowa athletic director, Coach Elliott, had called me into his office and said the NFL did not have all the paperwork they needed. That afternoon I had to scramble to fill out the formal petition to enter the draft and ship it by overnight mail to the NFL office. It wasn't until the next afternoon— the day before the draft—that I got official notification that I was indeed eligible. It was routine paperwork, but it had to be done. It almost wasn't.

"What else could go wrong?" I wondered to myself.

Just a few minutes after my dad called, the phone rang again. It was about 11:45 by this time.

"Jonathan, this is Les Miller. I'm the player personnel director with the Kansas City Chiefs."

"How are you today, Mr. Miller," I said, as coolly as I could but knowing this phone call was more serious.

"Fine. I just wanted to let you know that if you are still available, there is a chance we will take you with our second round pick."

Finally, I had something that almost seemed solid.

"That'll be fine with me," I said, wondering what it might be like to go to Kansas City.

This time, when I got off the phone, I let a little smile show. My roommates were begging to know every word Les Miller had said. We had determined since Dave Kendall's call that the Chiefs had the fourteenth pick. So they immediately began calculating when the Chiefs' turn would come up. It seemed as if it should be within the next hour.

For the first time that day, I let myself start getting excited. Still I made sure no one else could tell.

I kept playing down the Les Miller call, emphasizing that he didn't say for sure the Chiefs would draft me. They might be thinking about drafting me, I said, but so many things can happen. They could change their minds; another player could end up being available that they assumed another team would pick. It wasn't time to celebrate yet. But I was reasonably sure it wouldn't be long now.

I thought back on a conversation from the night before around our kitchen table. The four of us—Chuck, Mike, Hap, and me—were remembering how when we were kids we used to watch with awe the big-time college teams play on television on Saturday. Then, a few years went by and we became the ones the little kids were watching. Then as college players we would watch the pro games on Sunday, wondering if we would be good enough to join them one day. My day had come to find out, and they were all giving me a hard time about it.

"Well, Johnny, tomorrow's the day," Hap had said. "You're going to be up with the big boys." He was always egging me on. "And you're going to get your butt knocked off now."

I teased them back. "Yeah but at least I won't be broke anymore."

The four of us who had moved into this apartment together for my last semester had all come in as freshmen together. The bond of friendship among us was strong, and I knew I would really miss them.

They were genuinely excited for me. The way they had been bouncing around the apartment all morning, it seemed as if they were more excited than I was.

## 'The Call'

At 12:50 p.m., a little more than an hour after Les Miller's call, the phone rang again.

"Hello."

"Hello, is this Jonathan Hayes?"

"Yes it is."

"Jonathan, this is Barbara Harrington of the Kansas City Chiefs. . . ."

Before she finished introducing herself, I heard someone blast through the front door of the apartment building, nearly tearing the door off the hinges. He bolted up the stairs in three leaps and flung the apartment door open.

"YOU GOT DRAFTED!" It was Nick, who had made it across several blocks from his girlfriend's apartment where he had heard the announcement on television. He started hugging Hap, Mike and the others who were there. They were swinging their arms around, exchanging high-five's.

I frantically motioned to them to be quiet.

". . . I'd like to congratulate you. The Kansas City Chiefs have selected you with their second-round pick."

"Thank you very much," I said, straining to hear over the shouting and hand slapping going on around me. Chuck had come charging in just a few seconds behind Nick. Others had followed.

"I have Coach Mackovic and Jim Schaaf on the other line, and they would like to speak with you."

John Mackovic was the Chiefs' head coach at the time, and Jim Schaaf was the general manager. Jim Schaaf spoke for only a few moments, simply welcoming me to the team. Then Coach Mackovic told me that the Chiefs selected me not only for my athletic ability but also because of the kind of person I was. They asked if I could come to Kansas City immediately for a media session that afternoon and some initial meetings. That wouldn't be possible, I said, because of some class work I had to finish up. I did have a speech to give and a paper to turn in the next day, but the truth was that I did not want to miss the evening of celebration with my friends.

When I hung up the phone, the apartment exploded into utter chaos. By now, people were pouring through the door, and each new arrival would stimulate a new round of shouts and cheers, high-five's and hugs. Someone grabbed the champagne and began popping corks. The party was on.

## Draft Celebration

"How in the heck did you get over here so fast?" I shouted to Nick, amid the laughing and screaming. "You were here almost as soon as I picked up the phone."

The Chiefs had made me the forty-second overall pick in the draft. I ended up being the first tight end and the first Iowa player drafted. The Giants, who had called me earlier, did draft a tight end, Mark Bavarro, but not until the fourth round.

Amid the enthusiastic partying, the phone kept ringing with well-wishers. My parents, who were as elated as anyone, had their own draft day party going in Pittsburgh. My brother Jay called, and he began preparing me for what would come as I tried to break into pro ball. He shared some of his experiences from trying to make the Detroit Lions and Washington Redskins squads a few years before. He had ended up playing one year for the Michigan Panthers and two years for the Memphis Showboats in the United States Football League before the league folded. His experiences provided valuable lessons for me, and his excitement was contagious as he speculated about my chances with the Chiefs.

After an hour or so of celebration, I placed a call at the agreed upon time for a telephone news conference with Kansas City reporters. They asked the standard questions to which I gave fairly generic replies. "Man is it loud there," one reporter commented before his question. "Are you having a party or something?"

I smiled and looked around at the crowd that now filled the apartment wall to wall. "Yeah, I have a few friends over."

We kept getting reports about the other Iowa players; we were all pulling for them to get picked soon as well. Owen Gill, who had called to congratulate me on my pick, became the fifty-third pick overall, going in the second round to Seattle. George Little went in the third round to the Miami Dolphins. Both came over and joined the party at our place.

The anxious wait had finally ended. A new dream would soon begin.

# CHAPTER
## 4

# WELCOME TO
# THE NFL

**N**ear Kansas City I pulled off Interstate 35 and followed the signs to William Jewell College, where the Chiefs would gather for the 1985 version of the preseason ritual known as training camp. After several blocks, I spotted the sign that read "Kansas City Chiefs ...."

Before checking in with the team officials, I wanted to drive into the facility and scope out the fields that would introduce me to my professional future. I pulled up in the adjoining parking lot and sat quietly for a few minutes, gazing out the car window at the two practice fields that sit side by side at the crest of a hill on the school's campus. The summer sun was setting behind the trees on the far side of the fields, its rays extending toward me across the rich, green grass. With my college days behind me, this scene marked a new beginning in my football career. This peaceful grassland in front of me would soon become a violent battleground where only the strongest would survive. Could I become one of the survivors?

This was my fourth trip to Kansas City. I had come into town in April earlier that year, the day after the draft, to do some interviews with the local press and meet with the coaching staff. Since the pre-season spring mini-camp was to start the following week, I decided to stay and use those few days to get familiar with the city. Mini-camp was the first chance to meet the other draft picks and get some work in with the position coach. We got copies of our play books and began to learn the offensive scheme.

After the spring mini-camp, I had returned to Iowa City and finished my finals. Clearly life was immediately different. Though I had not yet signed with the Chiefs, that did not stop me from spending the money I expected sometime within the next several weeks. The first thing I did was walk into a car dealer, fix my eye on a big, champagne-colored Oldsmobile Toronado, and offer $18,000. Even though I didn't have a nickel to speak of, the dealer let me drive it away with only a promise of a cash payment later. At the end of June, after I signed, I cut him a check for the full amount. Yes, life had changed.

## Training Camp Begins

Nevertheless, though I had already begun to enjoy the benefits of a healthier bank account, that still didn't mean I would make the team. It didn't mean those paychecks would keep coming.

Orientation meetings filled most of the first day of regular training camp. It wasn't until the following day that we put on pads and had our first contact drills. At that time there was no limit to the number of players a team could bring into training camp, so I was out there with more than 60 guys, mostly the rookies and younger players who had not had much playing time, and a few guys who had been injured the year before. Right away, the hitting was intense, all of us trying to demonstrate to the coaching staff that we belonged at this level.

Because Ethan Horton, the Chiefs first pick in that year's draft, had not signed yet, I was the highest draft pick in camp. That meant the reporters focused on me as the newcomer. Each day I would face a barrage of questions about the direction the team was going, where I would fit, the transition from college to pro football. Of course, I offered the kinds of answers I knew they were seeking. The truth was, though, I was concentrating on only one thing: making the team.

That first camp was the most draining period of my entire career. The two-a-day workout schedule in the summer heat was physically exhausting, but I never slacked up, knowing the coaching staff was continually evaluating my performance. The mental strain was intense as well because as a new player I had to memorize all the plays, the tight end blocking assignments and pass routes, and the team's terminology.

The coaches do all they can during camp to make sure you eat, sleep, and think of football and football only. But I had to pay attention to more than football. I also had to continually monitor my sugar level and make sure it remained within an appropriate range. In the previous months during my off-season Iowa City routine, I had learned what it would take to keep my levels stable. But now the conditions had changed dramatically. Coaches and staff were in charge, and I had to fit in with their program. Workouts were so physically demanding that I had to learn all over again how my body would react. The team provided all the meals, so while most guys loaded their plates full of anything they found on the table, I had to pick and choose according to how the foods would affect me. The rigorous schedule, however, did not leave open long blocks of time to evaluate how I was feeling and make adjustments.

I was able to load up on calories enough before the workouts to keep my sugar levels within a reasonable range. When I started feeling low, I would grab a piece of fruit or a couple of graham crackers, or swallow some Gatorade. It helped that before the final game at Iowa, I had been on a two-a-day practice schedule. Although it wasn't as grueling as this pro camp, I had at least had a chance to experience how my body reacted to intense exertion twice a day.

Throughout those several weeks, I had to keep working, keep pushing, keep performing. I ended up exhausted but from the normal strain of training camp not because of my diabetes.

When the veterans arrived, they altered the training camp atmosphere somewhat, bringing a little relief. They knew better how to pace themselves since they knew the routine, and we rookies could follow their lead. They could anticipate particular drills and know how much energy to reserve. They were also far more relaxed with the coaches. Rather than the respectful "Coach Mackovic" that I would invariably use to address the head coach, the old veterans would shout, "Hey, John," despite his preference for greater formality. The veterans' perspective was that we were all men on the field, both players and coaches—no formal titles necessary. We weren't in college anymore.

"What are you doing, Rook?" Henry Marshall, a veteran wide receiver, would ask when I would address the coach as a dignitary. That wasn't the way it was done, he explained. Henry was the elder statesman among the group of receivers that I fell in with that included Carlos Carson, J.T. Smith, Willie Scott, Stephone Paige, Walt Arnold, and Anthony Hancock. These were fun-loving, light-hearted guys. When it came to work on the field, though, they were all business.

"If you're in our group," Henry told me, "you work." He told me not to worry as much about memorizing every play as giving 100 percent on the field. The coaches figured you could learn the plays eventually, he said, but if you won't put out maximum effort they won't want you. Advice like that helped me survive.

Comic relief came from Anthony Hancock. We called him "Space"; you never quite knew what he might do or say next. One day during camp, we were working on techniques for getting past the defensive backs on pass routes when they were trying to hold us up on the line of scrimmage. Generally, the receiver will fake one way and go hard the other way to throw the back off balance. Anthony lined up one time, took a quick step to the side, then spun around in a complete circle, like a ballerina performing a dainty pirouette. Sure enough he got across the line—the defender had doubled over laughing.

"What are you doing, Anthony?" Coach Williamson, the receiver and tight end coach, would say when he did things like that.

"Just looking for a new way to get the job done, Coach," he would say, glancing over at us with a smirk to see if we were appreciating the entertainment.

That summer in 1985 was particularly hot. Radio weather reports warned daily to beware of heat stroke. Of course that didn't stop our coaches from pushing us through rigorous workouts. The hotter I got and the more fluids I would lose through perspiration, the more I had to grab for the Gatorade to keep my blood sugar level up.

The veterans would try to let their sentiments about the heat be known to the coaches.

"Hey, Hawkeye," Kenny Kremer shouted to me across the practice field one day, using my most common nickname. "Would your mother let your dog out in heat like this?" Fuzzy, the name we knew him by, was making sure Coach Williamson could hear.

## Rookie Serenade

The first night the veterans were in camp, I learned that the National Football League fraternity has its own set of traditions, especially regarding rookie initiation. When we assembled in the cafeteria for dinner after our two full workouts in the 100-plus degree heat, the veterans started their call for the ceremonial rookie song. All I wanted to do was eat my dinner and get ready for the evening meetings. But since I was the highest draft pick in camp, they demanded that I take my position at center stage. Smiling and shaking my head, I stared down at my plate, hoping my embarrassment would satisfy them. No such luck. They continued their relentless campaign for their rookie serenade. Soon the whole room was staring at me, insisting that my performance begin.

"Show him how it's done, Ledge," somebody called out to Todd Blackledge, who had paid his dues as a first round draft pick two years before. So Todd, who actually can sing quite well, hopped up on the chair and opened the evening entertainment.

"I'm Todd Blackledge. . . from Penn State. . . and I play quarterback. . ." he opened, like a rhythm and blues performer. The guys began backing him up with clapping. Then, keeping with the same beat, he opened his song:

"I got sunshine. . . ." he started in, sweeping his arms dramatically through the air. The guys started hooting and cheering, egging him on. He played it up even more, swaying back and forth and cradling an invisible microphone, spinning around to spread his entertainment across the whole room.

As he finished his rendition of the popular song,

the room rumbled with applause, which soon led into a chant for more—only this time from me. Once again, every head in the room turned my way.

"Oh, please, God, no," I mumbled to myself, covering my face with my hands. If I could have crawled out through a hole in the floor, I would have. The beads of sweat were breaking out on my forehead; my body temperature was climbing by the moment, as if a huge, hot spotlight were glaring on me. There was no way out.

"All right. All right." Begrudgingly, I stepped up onto a chair. Guys dragged their chairs to the middle of the room, clearing an open area for my personal stage. Everyone started clapping.

"And we don't want no college fight song, either," someone shouted, sealing off the easiest escape route for the rookies. They wanted some popular tune. I tried desperately to think of a song I knew the words to. Finally I thought of one.

Following Todd's example, I started with what I supposed was the required introduction:

"I'm Jonathan Hayes. . . from the University of Iowa. . . and I play tight end. . . ." I tried to modulate the words to keep up some kind of regular rhythm. Then I started my song:

"Under the boh-ahrd walk, we were having some fun. . . ." Todd's song had been right on key. My notes must have strayed a little off, judging from the response.

"Booo. . . . Boooo. . . ." But they wouldn't let me quit.

"Under the boh-ahrd walk. . . down by the sea—ee—ee—. . . ."

My reprieve arrived before I made it very far into the song. To my great relief, all heads turned toward the door where a new face had just walked in. It was none other than Ethan Horton, the number one pick, who had just signed his contract and arrived at camp. As soon as he made his appearance, he became the target of the group assault. They suddenly lost interest in my impromptu nightclub act and started calling for Ethan to sing.

Greatly relieved, I got down off the chair, went over and got some ice cream, and settled back down, hoping to enjoy my dessert and let Ethan take over the entertainment. But I sensed someone staring at me. As almost everyone focused on Ethan, calling for his song, I looked over to find Lloyd Burruss, one of our defensive backs, pointing his finger at me. He let me know that I was by no means off the hook. "You still owe us one," he said.

Meanwhile, Ethan's resistance weakened, and he finally bowed to the group's demands. Instead of launching into a solo act, though, Ethan begged me to join him.

So we both ended up on adjacent chairs, performing for the elder brethren of the football fraternity an initiation rite I hoped I would never have to repeat. The clapping started up again, establishing a rhythm, and as a newly formed duet, we began our performance.

I knew my singing had been bad, but when I heard Ethan's voice, even I cringed. My notes may not have been precisely on key, but this guy was trying to reach for the sky and couldn't quite reach the treetops. The clapping began to subside, and as Ethan did his best Wayne Newton imitation, especially on the long, high notes, the groaning increased.

"Sit down, rookies," the judges finally proclaimed. "God, you're awful."

They made him practice during the rest of training camp. He needed it.

Since we were the highest draft choices in camp, Ethan and I roomed together at the training facility. It was a relief when I found out Ethan was familiar with diabetes. When he first saw me pull out my syringe to prepare for my insulin shot, he didn't flinch a bit. One of his family members, his grandmother I believe, had diabetes, and frequently Ethan had seen her inject her insulin.

## No Parking

The veterans also had a strict rule about parking places. No rookie was allowed to park in the spaces near the dormitory rooms. We could only use spaces at the bottom of the hill, then walk up. It didn't matter if there were empty spaces; they were off limits to rookies. Bob Olderman, a first-year offensive tackle, went to the lot after a meeting one day and couldn't find his car.

"We told you not to park up here," one of the guys said gruffly, glancing over to the others standing nearby and flashing them a quick smile. They had called a tow truck and had his car hauled away.

## Be Still, My Heart

Art Still, the Chiefs All-Pro defensive lineman, had held out that year and reported late to training camp. Before he arrived, I was warned that he was cut out of a slightly different mold.

At tight end, I would have to block him in our standard formation since he played left defensive end. At his first practice, I watched him shuffle onto the field. His shoes were untied, he had no pads in his pants, and he hadn't even buttoned his shoulder pads.

"Man, this guy must be tough," I thought.

In our first inside drill, when the offensive line and running backs go against the defensive linemen and linebackers, the play was a run right over Art. My job was to block him straight ahead. Coach Williamson told me to come off the ball hard and try to knock Art's head off.

Art called everyone "Cuz."

"Pssst, Cuz," he said quietly, as we each crouched down into our three-point stance. "If you come down on me hard, you're going to start a war."

I kept looking straight ahead and didn't say anything.

At the snap, I pushed off as hard as I could. My feet kept moving; I was snorting and grunting. Art barely budged. He was a big, powerful guy but his hands were especially strong. He had become known for his defense against the run.

"Psst, Cuz," he said, after the play. "We're not playing for real today. Rest yourself."

That's the same way he toyed with his opponents' minds in games, too. Few guys would survive even a few weeks in the league if they practiced as casually as he did. But when Sunday came, no one matched his intensity. He knew what it took to prepare himself. He knew his opponents and could anticipate their moves. But he was always a card on the field.

At key points in a game, when the home crowd would be on their feet clapping and guys would be trying to pump the team up, shouting, "Come on, let's go!" he would look at the self-appointed cheerleader and say something like, "Psst, Cuz, where we goin'?"

I roomed on the same floor in training camp as Art. One day I came into his room to find his sheets and blankets on the floor, his mattress on its side against the wall.

"I always sleep on the floor," he said, in response to my curious gaze.

## Monday Night Madness

Each Monday after meetings that year, the receivers would gather for dinner at a favorite restaurant. I was delighted one Monday when they asked me to come along. It seemed like a chance to get more comfortable with the group, perhaps fit in and become "one of the boys." So I settled in at the table with Henry Marshall, Carlos Carson, Willie Scott, J.T. Smith, and a few others.

Football players can eat. Each guy ordered a different appetizer, then several other items off the menu, not to mention the steady flow of beers that came from the bar. The waitress kept noting each item ordered, tacking it onto the growing tab.

When the plates were scraped clean and the mugs drained, Henry Marshall turned toward me. "Hey, Rook," he said, nodding toward the center of the table. "Get the bill."

My jaw dropped. "What?" I protested. "But . . . ."

Henry leaned over toward me. "If you complain," he said, "you'll never get to come again." Of course, the dinner group got a good laugh out of this.

That was the veterans' way of saying, "Welcome to the NFL." That part of my welcome cost me over $600.

## Playoff Appearance

During my first two years in the league, the Chiefs had moderate success, due in large part to the defense and special teams. In 1986, my second year, we made the playoffs by winning our last four games. In a game against Pittsburgh, a must-win game in the playoff race, the special teams nearly won single-handedly, with some help from the defense, but no help at all from the offense. Special teams blocked a field goal and a punt and took them both back for touchdowns. The offense had stunk up the field so badly that the coach named a special teams player, Boyce Green, offensive player of the game.

Frank Ganz—"Crash" we called him—had been brought in as assistant head coach with responsibility for special teams. "How are you, good man?" he would say to every guy on the field before practice, shaking his hand and patting him on the back.

Frank was not only personable but was also an incredible motivator. Guys would come to sit in on the special teams meetings just to hear his orations. Often, his vast knowledge of history and military leaders would provide the backdrop for his instructions about special teams play. We would be scratching our heads, listening to a discourse about Gingus Khan's tactics in surrounding a Mongol garrison. Sure enough, he would bring it around to his strategy for shutting down the San Diego kick return.

We lost in the first round of the playoffs in 1986 to the New York Jets. Rumors started circulating shortly after the season was over that the assistant coaches, including Frank and Walt Corey, the defensive coordinator, were not going to be back. They were popular with the players; we felt they helped make us a better team.

Also, we were concerned about the team's future. The offense was one-dimensional, purely a passing attack. "I don't care how many Heisman Trophy winners we have in our backfield," Coach Mackovic had said, "we're going to pass the ball 50 times a game." The players felt we needed a more balanced offense.

A few of us were called in for a meeting at Nick Lowery's house with Lamar Hunt, the Chiefs' owner, and Jack Steadman, the president. At that meeting, we voiced our viewpoint that Frank and Walt were assets; we wanted them back next year. Later that day, I heard shocking news. John Mackovic had been fired. A few days later, Frank was the new head coach. That had certainly not been the move we were pushing for. We simply had not wanted to lose two good assistant coaches.

# Strike One

We started the 1987 campaign with enthusiasm. Frank was definitely a player's coach, far more personable than John Mackovic. With all its bright hopes, though, that season was gutted by a strike. Rather than the Chiefs progressing with the rebuilding program, the replacement players, as the league so respectfully called the players who took our place on the field during the strike—they were "scabs" to us—came in and managed to lose every game they played.

We seemed to have a scab-ball soap opera unfolding at Arrowhead Stadium that drew the attention of the entire nation. Each day as we prepared to set our picket lines, we would try to identify which gate the replacement players were coming in, so we could let them know how we felt about what they were doing.

The first day of the strike, we gathered in front of the Arrowhead offices, trying to anticipate the route of the scab bus. Bill Maas had been out hunting early that morning with Paul Coffman and Dino Hackett. As Bill turned his pickup truck into the parking lot, reporting for picket duty, Paul and Dino poised in the bed of the truck holding shotguns. Of course, cameras were rolling, and their stunt, which we all thought was hilarious, became the leading national news of the strike. That night, America watched as a Chiefs posse "hunted" the Arrowhead scabs.

Another day, Otis Taylor, former great wide receiver for the Chiefs who still worked with the club, drove in with a replacement player. I had just finished my early morning shift on the picket line and left for home, so it was the next shift that greeted Otis. He had noticed that someone had purposefully scratched up a replacement player's car, probably with a key or some other sharp object. Understandably, he got perturbed. He made the mistake, though, of accusing the players.

The guys explained that they had nothing to do with it, pointing out that there were several people around, any one of whom could have done this deed. Crowds would form around us whenever we were picketing—some sympathetic onlookers, some reporters, some sightseers. Of course, we couldn't control what some individuals in that crowd did.

Somehow in the heat of the dispute, Jack Del Rio and Otis Taylor started exchanging punches and wrestled each other to the ground. Again, the cameras had been rolling. That evening, network viewers, including my mother in Pittsburgh, were treated to a show featuring the Chiefs players squaring off against their own Hall-of-Famer. It wasn't pretty.

Another incident in the unfolding Arrowhead soap opera—or situation comedy if you prefer—occurred when a guy, wanting to take his shot at getting on television, walked up to Gate A and started blasting us for disrupting the season. We listened patiently for awhile until he started getting a little too abusive for our taste. Standing nearby were Mike Bell, a defensive end; Rich Baldinger, an offensive lineman; and me. We walked over close to him, trying to persuade him to shut his mouth. The next thing we knew, the guy was rolling down the hill. I guess we might have given him a little shove.

That night my mother called and scolded me. "I know that was you," she said, describing one of the players she could see from the side on the nightly news.

Some of those replacement players caught on with the team, but as far as we were concerned they always carried a bright red "X" on their backs. They were fair game in practice, and we always made it a point to let them know they had not earned a legitimate spot in the football fraternity.

# Disjointed Seasons

That season was a bust. By the time we got the replacement players out of the way and we got back on the field, the season was lost. Our final record was an abysmal 4-11-1. We would have to wait till the following year.

Again, hopes were high in training camp before the 1988 season, which would be the first uninterrupted year under Frank Ganz and his staff. But again the year was frustrating. We competed hard but lost several close games and ended up at 5-11.

That was Frank's last chance, and the Chiefs management decided at that point to make wholesale changes in the organization.

It's no wonder to me that we did not win consistently during those first several years. I had four different offensive coordinators during my first five years in the league. About midway through each year, we would begin catching on to that offensive coordinator's scheme and start winning games. By that point, though, we would be out of contention. It takes time and practice to work together as an offensive unit, each player learning his assignments and getting a feel for what the guys next to him are going to do. So just as we would begin to gel as an offensive unit, we would be saying hello to a new head coach or a new offensive coordinator, or both.

When we heard the rumors after the 1988 season that perhaps the Chiefs were going to bring in Carl Peterson as general manager, our reaction was, "Here we go again."

Meanwhile Marty Schottenheimer had left Cleveland. It looked as if he were on his way to San Diego, but we knew Carl had been talking to him, courting him for the Kansas City job.

My family had an unusual connection with the

Schottenheimers. My mother went to the same high school Marty attended near Pittsburgh, and she spoke quite highly of Marty's dad.

But my brothers ran into a bit of a problem that involved Marty. He had attended college at the University of Pittsburgh with a neighbor of ours, Jim, and the two had remained good friends. One day my brothers were walking home when Jim pulled up and offered them a ride. Jeff, about 7 at the time, looked in the car to see not only Jim but another man, this one a stranger. Because my father had drilled us about never getting into a car with a stranger, Jeff turned down the ride. Jay, on the other hand, who was about 5, accepted. When Jay got home, he got a whipping from my dad for taking a ride with a stranger. That stranger was Marty Schottenheimer.

Ironically, nearly 30 years later, this stranger would be my head coach. We were glad to hear the news that Carl had signed him. It would be another round of changes, but Marty was a proven winner. We just hoped he would be here for awhile.

# CHAPTER 5

## "AT TIGHT END . . .
## NUMBER EIGHTY-FIVE. . ."

As usual, it was a year before Marty Schottenheimer's system worked its way through our minds and we began to perform consistently on the field. In 1990, Marty's second year, we ended up 11-5, and made our return to the playoffs. But we lost in the first round to the Miami Dolphins, a game we should have won.

In 1991, we began the year with as much focus as we had ever had since I had been a part of the organization. Marty is all business, and the primary business that concerns him is winning a world championship.

With our record at 8-5, we faced a key match-up with the San Diego Chargers. We had already beaten them earlier in the year in San Diego, but they had improved dramatically and had begun winning games. We knew it would be tough to beat them a second time. A win, though, would mean clinching a wild-card playoff spot, guaranteeing us a chance to avenge our previous year's first-round loss.

### Game Day
To give an idea of a typical game day for me in the National Football League, I'll give a blow by blow

description of my activities on the day of that San Diego game at Arrowhead Stadium on December 8, 1991.

## *Pregame*

7:40 a.m. Alarm sounds. I pull out my monitor and check my level. Take my first shot of the day as soon as I get up. Mix 25 units NPH, the longer-range-type insulin that helps break food down throughout the day, and 5 parts regular, which helps over the next several hours. Jump in the shower. Get dressed.

8:15 a.m. Eat my regular breakfast: two bowls of cereal, two pieces of toast, and a glass of cran-grape juice. That week I had been down with a cold. I was feeling better, but the doctor had prescribed some cough syrup, warning me to watch my blood sugar.

8:30 a.m. Leave house for Arrowhead. Not much traffic on Sunday morning. My mind is free to think about the game.

8:50 a.m. Arrive at stadium. Jump into the whirl-pool. Get dried off and go to see trainers. They tape my ankles and wrists. I pull on my socks and T-shirt.

9:30 a.m. Several guys gather for a chapel service. A Kansas City area Christian musician named Paul Clark conducts the service.

10:00 a.m. Chapel over. Put on pants and shoes. Ask equipment manager about field conditions to determine proper shoes. Talk to Pete Holohan, another tight end, about the game plan. We talk about some of the things their linemen might do and different situations that might develop. We had set up a line-blocking call that week in case the defense showed a certain formation; I would signal to John Alt to bring him over to help block the man in front of me. I sit and drink one of the high-carbohydrate drinks they have for us in the locker room. It tends to bump my sugar up a bit but it helps before the game. I figure the exertion during the game will even out my sugar level. Sometimes I'll let my level get up to 200 or 210 before a game. By the end of the game, it will usually get back down to 75 or 80.

10:20 a.m. I stop back in the training room. Deron Cherry is up on the training table. David Lutz comes in. They're kidding around about the George Foreman fight the night before.

10:30 a.m. Coaches have been coming in and out, saying things that come to mind. Some of the guys are getting stretched by strength coaches. I lay down on my back and put my legs up over a leather chair and lay my head back on the floor. It helps me stretch my back and just relax before the game. I continue talking with Pete off and on. Tim Grunhard, our center, always goes up early with his pads on to mess around and check the field. Today he came back with the report that it was fairly dry.

Pete went out looking for a girl who was supposed to be waiting for an autographed football and picture. Jim Everett, whom Pete played with before in Los Angeles, had met this woman at the Indianapolis 500, and she asked for a football with Jim's and Pete's signatures on it. Jim had signed it, then, when we played the Rams earlier that year, had passed it on to Pete to sign. Pete had held it in his locker for a couple of weeks, and he finally got a note from this lady asking where the ball was. So he had to go up and look around in the stands to find her. The arrangement was that she would hold up a sign that said, "For Pete Holohan." So he was wandering around the field looking up in the stands for this sign. He finally found her. We laugh about the ordeal, joking about how we have nothing else to be thinking about before the game but passing out autographed footballs.

Dave Redding comes through and shouts that it is nearly time for the specialists—that's the quarterbacks, receivers, kickers, kick returners, and long snappers—out on the field.

10:58 a.m. Specialists go out to field. That's my cue to head to the equipment room. Mike Davison, our equipment manager, helps me get my pads on. He also helps David Lutz, Bill Maas, Rich Baldinger, and John Alt. Our shirts are tight over our pads, so we always have Mike help us. Of course any of the equipment managers could help, but we always have Mike do it. You do something one way for so long, you get a little superstitious.

11:00 a.m. Troy Sadowski, a backup tight end, and I go out for a lap around the field to start getting warmed up. The running backs go out at the same time. I run right over to Al Saunders, wide receivers coach, and he throws me several passes, trying to prepare me for pass-catching situations that might come up during the game.

11:10 a.m. The linemen and linebackers come out on the field, and the entire team gathers in one end zone. We do "take-offs," where we run up to the middle of the field where another coach is standing. He says, "Go again," and we turn around and run back to the end zone where we started. Then we all line up and stretch. The receivers run pass routes with the quarterbacks.

11:20 a.m. We run the pat-and-go drill where the quarterbacks slap the ball, drop back a few steps, and fire the ball to the receivers who are running their patterns. Meanwhile the interior linemen, linebackers, and defensive backs are doing their separate drills.

11:25 a.m. Coach Redman shouts "On air." We begin the "on air" drill, which means we start running the pass routes hard. After a few repetitions, we switch ends of the field, so we get accustomed to the conditions on both ends.

11:35 a.m. We run 7 on 7, or "pass skeleton." The

receivers, running backs, and tight ends line up against the linebackers and defensive backs. We practice routes but without any serious contact.

11:40 a.m. Marty calls the entire team together to run a series of plays—two from the 35-yard-line, two from the 20, and two from the two-yard-line. The kicking team runs through one punt, and Nick Lowery kicks one field goal.

11:46 a.m. We head back to the locker room. Guys are taking care of whatever they need to do to get ready for the game: going to the bathroom, getting taped up, threading shoestrings, toweling off perspiration, changing clothes and equipment. It's a nice day so we don't need to get coats. Sometimes I check my sugar level with a monitor at this point. But today I'm feeling good, so I don't think there is any need.

11:55 a.m. Everyone circles around Marty and says "The Lord's Prayer" together.

11:57 a.m. We file out of the locker room and line up in the tunnel for introductions.

11:58 a.m. The announcer is introducing the starting offense for this game, so I listen to the names of the guys ahead of me. When my turn comes, I take a moment to adjust my helmet and start my trot through the cheerleaders toward the middle of the field. "... At tight end, number 85, Jonathan Hayes. . . . " The applause starts the adrenaline pumping. It's tough to tell sometimes whether the anxiety I feel before a game is pre-game adrenaline, just like everyone else is feeling, or if it's a result of low blood sugar. The two conditions feel about the same. If I can't get myself calmed before a game, I'll go ahead and pull out my monitor to check.

11:59 a.m. Once on the field, I run straight to Bud Epps, our trainer. He throws me a towel, I wipe my face, and he puts a single line of "black eye," the black powder that helps deflect the glare from the sun, under each eye. Then, like always, I rub his head. I wouldn't feel right starting a game without going through that routine.

12:00 p.m. I line up next to Mike Bell for the National Anthem. Bud stands next to him on the other side. After the final note, I trot back to the bench and kneel down to pray briefly. Then I'm ready to play.

### First Quarter

12:01 p.m. We win the toss. I take the field with the kickoff return unit. I'm glad I'm on kickoff return because you get to go out a start banging heads right away. You don't have to wait until the first play from scrimmage. They kick the ball to our far left. We run "wedge on the ball," a very basic return. I had to run fairly far across the field to get to Bill Jones, who sets the wedge. We came right up the middle of the field. I hit my guy in the ribs and throw him to the ground. It always feels good to make that first contact.

The offense takes the field. We start moving the ball but get stopped short of a first down. After our punt, San Diego starts moving steadily. After a long drive that takes up most of the first quarter, they score the first touchdown of the game and take the lead 7-0.

### Second Quarter

12:40 p.m. Our offense starts driving, but our quarterback Steve DeBerg throws an interception on an out pattern. The defender takes his return down the sideline all the way for a touchdown to make the score 14-0. The "boobirds" come out in force.

### Halftime

1:20 p.m. We look at a series of still photos to evaluate their defensive sets. Coaches emphasize that we have to make sure our quarterback doesn't get hit. We talk over a couple of the blocking schemes we had trouble with.

Some of the guys show some frustration, but we keep our heads. We are determined not to let San Diego come into our home field and take away a chance for us to get into the playoffs.

### *Third Quarter*

1:40 p.m. Marty starts Mark Vlasic. I'm reminded of our days at Iowa together. Mark takes the offense down the field. His first pass is directly over the middle to me. I run a hook pattern, just far enough downfield for a first down. That completion, from one Iowa boy to another, helps Mark get his confidence going, as well as keeping the drive alive. We get far enough downfield for Nick to come in and kick a field goal to bring the score to 14-3. Then the defense steps up strong. Dino Hackett comes blitzing right up the middle, forcing the quarterback to throw an errant lateral pass. Derrick Thomas picks it up at the San Diego 1 yard line. On our first offensive play, the back runs right behind left tackle John Alt and me. I don't get a great initial surge. But we keep our feet moving and hold our guys up. Billy Jones, the fullback, leads the play. Barry Word gets the ball and hits the line of scrimmage. We all press hard into the defenders, enough to allow Barry to get into the end zone. The score moves to 14-10.

### *Fourth Quarter*

2:20 p.m. The key play in the quarter is a completion to Harvey Williams, which comes on a bit of a trick play. He sneaks back toward the left sideline while Pete Holihan, me, and the rest of the receivers run patterns to the right side of the field. Harvey ends up virtually alone in the end zone. Touchdown. We take the lead 17-

14. But San Diego uses the three minutes remaining on the clock to get into field goal range and tie the score.

### *Overtime*

3:10 p.m. Since the game is going longer than usual, I take a moment to think whether my blood sugar might be getting low. I hadn't eaten since 8:15 this morning, but I feel fine.

We win the toss again and get the ball first. But we can't score on our first possession. The special teams do a great job. Brian Barker punts the ball out of bounds on the San Diego 4. When we get the ball back, we get closer but still stay out of field goal range because of a penalty. Brian punts again. This time, Todd McNair bats the ball back just as it is heading into the end zone. Charles Washington catches it and sets it down on the 1 inch line before he falls into the end zone. Then Lonnie Marts kneels down and carefully downs it. The defense keeps them in the hole, nearly getting a safety and ending the game right then. San Diego has to punt from the back of their end zone. Troy Stratford returns it inside the San Diego 40. On the first play from scrimmage, running back Barry Word breaks through the line and past the linebackers, and the defensive backs can't catch him until he's to the 1 yard line. It was one of those perfect plays where everyone got clean blocks, just like we draw it up on the blackboard. My job was to seal off the defensive end so he couldn't circle around the backside to reach the running back. Rather than risk the turnover on a running play, Marty right away sends Nick Lowery in to kick the chip-shot field goal. The game is over. Chiefs 20, San Diego 17.

### *Post-Game*

3:35 p.m. It was a hard-fought game, and the Charger players have been our enemies for the last 60-

plus minutes. But once the game is over, I look around for friends. We share a lot of ties with other players in the league. Some are former Chiefs teammates. Some are fellow Iowa Hawkeyes. And some are players I have played against for so long that we have earned each other's respect.

Right away, I find Ronnie Harmon, a fellow Hawkeye. When we had played in San Diego, he arranged for some fried chicken to be waiting for me in the locker room after the game, so I had done the same for him today. I say hello to Kittrick Taylor, who had been with the Chiefs a couple of years before. I greet other guys who had become friends after playing against them for so long: Martin Bayless, one of their cornerbacks, who later would be signed by the Chiefs; Billy Ray Smith, an outside linebacker, and Bert Grossman, a defensive end, who I had been blocking on all day.

3:45 p.m. Once most of us make it to the locker room we gather again to say a prayer, and Marty makes a few comments. Then the linemen and tight ends congregate. We're like a herd of cattle hanging around together all the time. We talk about the plays that worked, the calls that were made. The better we know each other, the better we play. It's especially important for the linemen to talk because the line has to function as a unit.

There's a little extra excitement today because of winning a tough game and because the win clinches a playoff spot. After a few minutes, I sit down on the stool by my locker and relax, looking around the room, wondering which team we will face in the playoffs. The locker room is filling up quickly now. That happens when we're winning. In previous years, when we weren't as successful, it was so empty in the locker room you could hear an echo. Now pockets of reporters are crowding around lockers, grasping pencils and notepads and shoving tape recorders toward several guys' faces. Lamar Hunt stops by my locker and says hello and congratulations. He is always encouraging.

I walk back to the shower, stopping in the training room on my way. I make it a point to congratulate the guys on defense, especially the linemen and linebackers. We share a camaraderie because we all know what it is like in the trenches during a tough game like this one. I also step over to Steve DeBerg to encourage him after a tough day.

3:50 p.m. Now that I am winding down from the game, I feel like my blood sugars might be a little low, especially since we had to keep working hard through the overtime. I prick my finger and check my blood. It's at 107, which isn't bad. But that doesn't tell me whether the level is going up or down. I drink a soda to hold me over until I can get something to eat.

### *Evening*

4:15 p.m. On my way out of the stadium parking lot, I call my mom and dad from my car phone, like I do every Sunday after a game. Mom says she wore her "Hayes' Huddle" T-shirt under her dress to church that morning. They weren't able to pick this game up on their satellite, so I filled them in on some of the key plays.

6:15 p.m. Derrick Thomas had planned a dinner get-together for the team at Garozzo's, an Italian restaurant in downtown Kansas City. When I arrive, I check my sugar level again because most of the guys are watching the Buffalo-Los Angeles Raider game, and I know we won't eat till it is over. My sugar level is 127, so I know I will be all right until dinner. I go in the bathroom and take my second insulin shot of the day, then join the other guys to watch the game. We eat dinner around 6:45. I hang around for awhile, then around 8:30 head over to the Ritz-Carlton Hotel, where Nick Lowery is hosting a cocktail party. After about 30 minutes there I take off for home.

9:30 p.m. Within 15 minutes of arriving home, I'm in bed for the night.

## Playoff Progress

We got as far as the second round of the playoffs in 1991, beating the Los Angeles Raiders in the first round but then losing the following week to Buffalo, who would go on to the Super Bowl. The second-round appearance marked progress over the previous year, but was not nearly enough success to satisfy Marty or the rest of the team.

Not only did we begin the year in 1992 with focus, but also with confidence. This team seemed to be gaining momentum, and we came into training camp aiming for the Super Bowl. The biggest question mark coming into camp was at the quarterback position. We had signed Dave Krieg in the off-season, and we were hoping that he could add another dimension to our offense.

While we had had some success during the regular season, beating some outstanding teams like Washington, Philadelphia, and San Diego twice, we also faltered in a few games that we should have won. Early in the year, John Elway, the Bronco quarterback, had brought the Broncos back in the final couple of minutes in Denver after we had been ahead by nearly two touchdowns.

We faced the final regular season game at Arrowhead with a 9-6 record, needing to beat Denver to clinch a playoff spot. The game started slowly with neither team taking charge. After punting on our first couple of possessions, the offense finally started moving. Dave

Krieg tossed me a flare pass. It was a little low, but I was able to reach down, grab it with one hand, and pull it up to my side. I turned upfield and picked up 7 or 8 yards for a first down. The drive continued downfield, and we got our first points on the board with a field goal.

The defense did a great job of controlling Denver. The linemen and linebackers were all over John Elway and never gave him a chance to do much damage.

In the second quarter, we pushed the ball down close to the Denver goal line. We called a play that sent me out on the pattern with the outside receivers. Dave found me in the end zone, and I caught my first touchdown pass of the year.

Later, we were near their goal line again, and Dave called a run-pass option. He rolled out to the right and watched the cornerback to see if he came up to defend the run or stayed back to cover the pass. Meanwhile, I curled around near the back of the end zone. When I saw the cornerback begin charging toward Dave, I figured he would toss me the ball. He threw it to the edge of the end zone. I was careful to plant both feet in bounds, then lean over to grab the ball. It was my second touchdown catch of the game, the first time I had ever had two in one game, and my fourth catch overall that day.

We beat Denver in that final regular season game and secured a playoff spot for the third consecutive year. In the first round we faced San Diego, a team we had beaten twice earlier in the year though they had snuck by us to win the division. They were a much improved team, and we knew they would be tough. Unfortunately, the 1992 season ended with a disappointing first-round playoff loss to the Chargers. The quest for a world championship would have to continue.

# Doctor of My Own Body

Over the years, most of my teammates have known about my diabetes. I don't broadcast it, but I don't hide it either. The trainers know to ask me periodically how I'm feeling and to offer regular shots of Gatorade. But for the most part it is up to me to make sure that I take care of myself on and off the field so that I'm prepared to practice and play hard every week.

Like anyone else, I like to feel good before I play. My challenge is not completely unlike any other player. We all have to be sure that in general we get enough rest, eat well, and stay in shape. I just have to pay closer attention to my body than anyone else.

But after several years of practice, I have learned to be a reasonably skilled doctor of my own body. Of course, I work closely with my own physician to maintain proper control. Occasionally my insulin level needs to be adjusted, or a situation will come up that we need to discuss together. But for those of us with diabetes, the day to day issues of monitoring blood sugar levels, eating properly, getting exercise, and taking medication fall to us. It has now become second-nature to pay attention to what my body is telling me. I really don't have to think consciously about my blood sugar levels too much, though it's always in the back of my mind. I have learned to read certain "signals" that tell me if my levels are a little off.

Sometimes, for example, I can tell that my urine gets a little light. That's a signal that there is sugar in it, which means the sugar is discharging through my kidneys and I will need to bring my blood sugar level down. Other times my joints will ache, which tells me my sugar level is getting high.

If I suspect that I'm low or high, or if I can't tell for sure by the way I feel, I'll pull my meter out, prick the end of my finger to get a couple of drops of blood on a test strip, and check my sugar level.

If I get low before a game, I'll drink some Gatorade, grab an orange, or eat some of the crackers or bread that I keep in my locker. For away games, I'll make sure to grab a few extra rolls from the pre-game meal and drop them in my bag so I know I have something to eat if I need it. If my sugar level gets high, I'll go in and climb on the exercise bike to try to bring it down some, and I'll drink a lot of water, which also helps.

Monitoring my physical condition has become like part of my playbook, a normal part of my world.

The regular season provides a tight structure of practices, workouts, and games. That structure helps me to maintain a fairly regular routine of eating and exercising. During the season, I have to bump up my calorie intake to as much as 6,000 to 7,000 calories a day just to keep my blood sugar levels in the normal range. Of course, those calories are spread out over several meals and snacks throughout the day.

Irv Eatman, a good friend and former teammate, owns the record, in my judgment, for eating the largest quantity of food in one sitting. Once he gets started, he seems to keep eating forever. But that may be the only meal he'll eat in a day. If I followed that pattern, my blood sugar would shoot off the charts.

The off-season presents a different set of challenges. On the one hand, my workouts are lighter, so I'm not burning nearly as many calories, and I can cut back on quantity of food. But on the other hand, my day-to-day life is not nearly so structured, and sometimes I forget to eat enough. I spend much of my time working the horses that I train on my ranch south of Kansas City. I may grab a sandwich for lunch, thinking it will hold me over till dinner. But mid-afternoon, I'll sometimes catch myself getting low. My barn isn't like the Chief's training facility where there is Gatorade and fruit available all the time. So I'll have to get back to the house for a snack.

I've learned a few tricks over the years that help me avoid trouble. For instance, if I'm speaking at a banquet, I've learned that dinner often is not served until as late as 8:00 p.m. It isn't always easy to figure out how to get some food, especially if I'm supposed to be speaking to the group. My solution is to always eat a sandwich before I leave home.

## Sideline Support

During my first three years in the league, Walt Arnold was also a tight end with the team. After awhile I discovered that Walt had diabetes too. We would continually ask each other on the sidelines, "How are ya doin'?" "How ya feelin'?"

After the pregame meal, he would always take a napkin and wrap up several rolls to take along into the locker room. "Want one?" he would ask, offering me one of his slightly stale rolls. If I thought my blood sugar was getting a little low, I would take one.

We could also help each other out with supplies. Once, Walt ran out of syringes, and I was able to give him one of mine. Unfortunately, he blew out his knee in the '87 season and had to retire.

The next year I could have used Walt's help. We had flown to Los Angeles for a game against the Raiders. I discovered I was out of insulin and test strips, which I needed to check my blood sugar. I had gotten up a little later than planned, so the time was short. So while my teammates were lounging around the hotel, preparing for the game, I had to catch a cab and rush off to a pharmacy.

In my haste, I had failed to check my wallet. When it came time to pay for the supplies, I found only $45. That would be enough to pay the pharmacist. But what about the cab fare?

"Great," I thought. "I'm stuck in the heart of Los Angeles with no way to get back to the hotel." I hoped the cab driver would show some understanding. As soon as he pulled up to the hotel, I assured him I'd be right back. Fortunately, some of the guys were in the lobby, so I borrowed enough to pay the $20 fare. Ever since, I have made sure to have enough supplies with me, especially when we're on the road.

## Caught in the Act

In my second year in the league, Irv Eatman, an offensive tackle, and I roomed together after each of our original roommates had been cut from the team. After we got settled in our hotel room before our first road game, Irv asked if I wanted to get some dinner.

"Sure, let me take my medicine, and I'll be ready to go," I said, heading for the bathroom. As I pulled out my syringe and began measuring out the proper dosage of insulin, he paraded into the bathroom and started pleading with me, playfully.

"Don't do it, Johnny. Don't do it," he pleaded. His slight smirk showed he was razzing me. Once he got started, he kept getting more and more dramatic, as if only he stood between me and a deadly drug overdose. "It's not worth it, Johnny!"

He knew I had diabetes, but it was the first time he had seen me prepare for an injection. He took full advantage of the opportunity to harass me, and both of us ended up laughing hysterically. He continued his act on through dinner, telling all the guys the sad story about how I had gotten caught up on drugs and that he had interrupted me while I was shooting up. We were still laughing about that bathroom scene years later.

Actually, I'm glad the guys on occasion razz me about my diabetes. I don't want them treating me with kid gloves, afraid that bringing up the subject of my diabetes will somehow bother me. My greatest fear is that my peers will misunderstand my condition and feel pity for me. I don't want to be treated one bit differently because I have to deal with a serious disease.

With the coaching staff and management, I don't have to worry much about being treated differently. In my business, the only way to stay employed is to keep producing. They watch continually to evaluate performance, and I'll never get any reprieve from the demands on the field because of diabetes. If I lose the ability to knock the guy across the line on his backside, I'm history. We all understand the rules that govern this game.

## Do Unto Others

I also run across situations that give me a chance to treat others who face the effects of a disease or disability the way I want to be treated. During the offseason in 1992, I played in a celebrity golf tournament that Jan Stenerud helps organize to benefit a charity. The event coordinator pointed me toward the 10th tee, where I would join up with my foursome for the day. I greeted my partners, two ladies and another man. After watching the ladies tee off, I noticed immediately that the man was struggling to bend down, plant his tee in the grass, and balance his golf ball on it. Once he got the ball teed up and cocked his club back, I noticed that his hips barely moved and his knees bent only slightly. Using mostly his arms and upper body, he let loose a swing. Despite the awkward movements, he connected solidly with the ball and sent it well down the fairway.

This was one of those moments when I had to make a decision. If I ignored his obviously impaired condition, it would be on my mind for the next 18 holes.

From observing his movements, I was reasonably sure that the man had a prosthesis in place of one of his legs. If I said nothing, I would not be able to talk with him or even look at him without wondering what happened to him. My mind was dreaming up potential scenarios to explain the damage to his lower body. Was it a birth defect? Was it an accident? Was it a temporary condition, or permanent? Was it caused by a disease? In this situation, it seemed appropriate to ask.

"How did you lose your leg?" I asked, matter-of-factly.

"Motorcycle accident," he responded without showing even the slightest discomfort with the question.

After that, we were able to go on to the next hole and the several that followed talking about various things, without my mind being tied up with questions about his condition. I didn't see him as a man with an artificial leg; in my eyes he was just a man playing golf for a charity.

Most people with disabilities will not be offended by questions about their condition. Avoiding the subject usually only adds to the awkwardness. Of course, the subject of a person's disability should be approached sensitively and respectfully. But it is generally helpful to step out of our ignorance and learn about the conditions other people face.

I don't want diabetes to form a barrier between me and the people I meet. I don't want my friends to be intimidated by the procedures I go through. Ignorance about diabetes, though, or any disease or unusual physical condition, can be a substantial obstacle. The solution I have found is information.

I would like people to know more about diabetes for a variety of reasons. First of all, people who have diabetes need to learn all they can to properly manage their condition. Too many people who are diagnosed fail to face the seriousness of the disease and tend to take lightly the potential complications—until, of course, they lose a limb, or their kidneys fail, or their vision deteriorates. Second, people who are at risk for getting diabetes need to know the symptoms to watch for. They can adjust their lifestyles now to minimize their risk for developing the disease later. Third, people who will never get diabetes can help those affected by it. Working together we can find a cure and continue to improve the lives of people affected by diabetes.

# CHAPTER 6

# GIVING BACK

The Chiefs 1990 preseason schedule included an August game with the Los Angeles Rams in Germany. The team chartered a flight, and gave the players a chance to take along one or two guests. My dad had been diagnosed the year before with Hodgkin's Disease. He'd had surgery in December, and he was trying to fight his way through to a recovery. When I heard about this game in Europe, I immediately knew which guests I wanted to bring along: my mom and dad.

My dad had been stationed in Germany in the 1950s, just a few years after the Germans poured the concrete in the Berlin Wall. Now that same wall was being torn down. It was an historic time, and I knew a return visit would be meaningful to my dad. I also thought the prospect of such a trip would boost his morale and motivate him to keep struggling to recover amid the strain of ongoing treatments.

When the time for the trip arrived, my dad was in good spirits, eager to make his first journey to Europe since his Army days. On the plane, rather than leaving him back in the less spacious seats for this eight-hour trans-Atlantic flight, I brought him up to the section where the players were sitting. He could stretch out across two seats. I went back and joined my mother, leaving my dad to relax with the players. Once in awhile, I would come up front to check on him; it was satisfying to see him enjoying himself with the other players. I appreciated the way the guys had taken to him and were incorporating him in their conversations and activities.

At first, I felt that it would be up to me to make sure my parents had a good time. Each day, though, when I returned from practice in the afternoons, they would be off somewhere sightseeing or exploring another restaurant. They were taking full advantage of this European visit and had no intention of sitting around in the hotel room waiting for me.

One night we got together with Chuck Long, who was then with the Rams backing up Jim Everett. My folks had always loved Chuck and were delighted to see him; our families had spent many afternoons together in Iowa City, munching on sandwiches and sipping sodas at tailgate parties after the Hawkeye games. After he left Iowa as a consensus All-America quarterback, Chuck spent his first four years in the league with Detroit. As it turned out, he spent a year and a half with the Rams. Later he would return to Detroit with a new offense and another chance to start.

The game was played on August 11, 1990, my 28th birthday, but the game on the field was not the best part of the trip for me. Watching my dad and mom enjoy themselves was my highlight; the smiles on their faces were my birthday present.

## Give and Take

One of the values my parents taught me was to give back. If you only take and take and take, my dad would tell me, the well will run dry. But if, on the other hand, you appreciate what you have and give some of yourself to others, you'll find a much deeper and longer-lasting satisfaction.

As I matured into adulthood, some of the first people I wanted to give to were my parents. Of course I know that I can never repay my parents for all they provided for my brothers and me. The trip to Germany, however, served as one of those opportunities to give back by providing an experience for my parents that they would value. It was satisfying.

As I have grown older, I have realized how great an impact my parents have had on my development as a person. They emphasized from my earliest years of childhood the importance of giving to others. Every Sunday, we were in church hearing more about caring for and respecting others. We emerged from childhood practicing an outlook on life that included showing concern for other people, especially those less fortunate than ourselves. My parents never demanded that we be perfect. They often recounted the Bible passage that says all of us fall short of God's perfect standard. But they taught us to aim high, to value other people, and to be the best people we could be.

A few years ago at a football camp that Bill Maas puts on, I found myself acting just like my dad. We went out for dinner at a restaurant, and one of the kids found something on his plate that he didn't like. "You better sit up there and eat," I said in my firmest voice. "You're not going to leave this table until you do." The words, even though they had come from my own mouth, shocked me. That could have been my father talking, I thought to myself. I suppose the greatest form of flattery is imitation.

## Community Life

During my first year at Iowa, a teammate introduced me to the kind of opportunity I frequently would have in the years to come. He asked me to come help with a special competition among mentally retarded children. I didn't know exactly what to expect, but I agreed to go. Even though I was a little apprehensive, the kids made me feel comfortable.

We taught them how to toss the football, and more importantly, how to score touchdowns and do a proper endzone dance. They loved the attention, and they openly expressed their love with hugs and smiles for everyone. They taught us something that day about unconditional love. They didn't seem to store up hurts or grudges toward anyone. The smiles on their faces and the look of innocence in their eyes affected me. I felt that I wanted to do more of this.

Once my professional career began, I had many opportunities to work with groups in the community helping people with special needs. It is tempting for an athlete to become isolated in the glamorous world of professional sports. I make a conscious effort to resist that temptation and to stay involved in people's lives outside my sport. I share the world with people who are hurting, kids who have special needs, parents who are struggling to make life work for themselves and their children. My parents showed me how caring makes a difference, so when I am in a position where I can help, I do.

I have had the opportunity to play in celebrity golf tournaments and basketball games, serve as celebrity bartender, and participate in benefit auctions for such groups as the United Negro College Fund, the Dream Factory, and the Harvesters Food Bank. I have had the opportunity to speak to thousands of junior and senior high school students in the Kansas City area about living positive lives, developing good study habits, and becoming better people through programs sponsored by such groups as Athletes in Action and the Boy Scouts.

For several years I participated in the Chiefs Corps, a program organized by the Chiefs and a corporate sponsor in which nine players would adopt an inner city school, meet several times a year with the students at an all-school assembly, and speak to the tenth grade English classes. The reward for the kids who kept their grades up was tickets to a Chiefs home game.

## Character Flaws

It's good to be able to use the platform of professional sports as a positive influence for young people. But athletes are just like everyone else—imperfect. While the public will see us helping in the community, they'll also see us when our flaws show.

A Kansas City schoolteacher called me one day in desperation and asked if I could help with one of her students. The kid was a good football player, she told me, and loved the Chiefs. But he kept getting into fights at school. I agreed to call him.

When we first spoke, I asked the boy how things were going at school. He explained about the recent fights. A kid had kicked a ball in his face in gym class, he said. As I started to reason with him about how he shouldn't fight, the realization struck me that I don't practice what I was about to preach. Here I was preparing a speech for a kid about not fighting when football fans across the country have seen me do more than my share of pushing and shoving and tough-talking in the heat of a football game.

I had to change my approach. I admitted to him that I fight too much. We both need to do better at controlling our tempers, I said. When I fight, I told him, I lose focus on what I'm trying to get accomplished. In my case, losing focus on blocking and catching passes could cost my team a game. Those are serious consequences. But for him the consequences could be even more serious, I said. He could get kicked out of school and lose his chance for an education.

We both need to be smarter, I told him, and stop fighting so much. To help motivate him, I promised him tickets to a home game and a trip out to my farm to ride horses—if he would stop fighting and do well in school.

## Diabetes Groups

Because of my diabetes, I have been particularly motivated to work with the American Diabetes Association and other groups that are working on finding a cure and improving treatment for diabetes. After all, every dollar I help raise at a celebrity waiters breakfast, a benefit auction, or a golf tournament may help bring my own cure, or at least improved treatment, that much closer. Funds raised also help make the summer camps for kids possible and help reach those who have diabetes but don't yet know it—an estimated 7 million Americans. The earlier the disease is detected, the better your chances of avoiding complications.

At times I have joined together with other athletes and celebrities who have diabetes to focus public attention on the disease. The International Athletes with Diabetes sponsored a forum in Washington, D.C., in 1990 that brought together Catfish Hunter, former pitcher for the Oakland Athletics; Kurt Frazier, former hockey player with the Minnesota North Stars; and Steven First, an actor who played Flounder in Animal House and Doc on St. Elsewhere. On another occasion I appeared in an educational video about diabetes management titled *Diabetes: A Positive Approach*, starring comedian Tom Parks. Each year I play in an

American Diabetes Association golf tournament in Kansas City that Freddie Patek has helped organize. Freddie is a former shortstop for the Kansas City Royals who also has diabetes.

Sometimes I get too much credit for these efforts; other times they go unnoticed. But I am not doing it for the pats on the back. The real reward has come from the friends I have met along the way. From these friends, kids with diabetes, mentally retarded athletes, and high school kids from the inner city, I have received far more than I have given. These kids face opponents as tough as any I've ever faced on the field, and they don't have the incentive of winning a Bowl game or turning pro to keep them going. But they do keep going.

## Summer Camps

Every year the American Diabetes Association sponsors summer camps for area kids who have diabetes. In the spring of 1986, after my first season with the Chiefs, the regional coordinator asked me to come join the kids for a couple of days.

My first day there, a young girl about 9 years old hopped up on my lap.

"How many shots do you take?" she asked, without hesitation. Of course I was accustomed to adults who tend to tiptoe carefully around the subject of my diabetes, assuming that discussing the disease openly will disturb me. Not this little girl. In this camp, nearly everyone had diabetes. They all spoke of insulin shots like most people speak of eating lunch—matter-of-factly. To these kids, taking shots, monitoring their blood sugar, and skipping sweets was a way of life, not an awkward subject to be avoided.

I chuckled at this little girl's forthrightness. "Two," I said.

She got a big smile on her face.

"Well, I take four," she said, "so I take more than you do." She lifted her chin triumphantly, as if she had just beaten me in a tough-guy contest.

This child's torso was barely bigger than my biceps, yet she felt she had proven greater toughness than I had—never mind how I have to go out and bang heads on the football field. I think she was right.

That little girl inspired me. This grade-school child was not feeling a bit sorry for herself because she had diabetes. Her face wasn't drooping as she spoke of her treatment. I think of myself as having courage to face 300-pound defensive linemen week after week. But she had the courage to take on a deadly disease and not let it get her down. She was living a normal life, proud of her own accomplishments—even proud of outdoing me!

In 1991, I had an opportunity to help a boy who was struggling during his first time at the American Diabetes Association summer camp. When I walked in for the first day of camp, several of the kids immediately crowded around and began their regular ritual: trying to tackle me. As usual, nine or ten kids were pulling on my arms and legs, determined to take me to the ground. I've gotten fairly good over the years at fending them off; the biggest one of them is about one-fifth the size of the linebackers and defensive linemen who are trying to do the same thing to me every Sunday from September to December.

In the midst of all this frivolity, I looked over and noticed one little boy, about 8 or 9 years old, sitting by himself. His cheeks showed a trail where tears had been falling. While most of the kids were wrestling, screaming, and shrieking with delight, he sat motionless, looking forlorn.

I went over to talk with him. This was his first year at camp, he told me, and he had just been diagnosed with diabetes a few months earlier.

"I just want to go home. . . . I just want to go home," he kept saying between sobs.

"Why don't you just hang out with me a little bit," I said, wishing for some way to soothe him. "Later if you still feel that way, we can call your mom." He consented but was not enthusiastic. He didn't care that I was a football player. It wouldn't have made a difference to him if I had caught 20 touchdown passes that season. He just wanted out of there.

It became clear to me that this was a crucial point in this little boy's life. If he could not get over the obstacle of being away from home now, it might be even more difficult for him next time. Camp is an opportunity for kids, often for the first time, to learn about managing their diabetes independently from their parents. It is a significant step for these kids to take.

We pulled out a letter from his mom and gave it to him to read. The counselors have all the parents write a letter to their child ahead of time for just such an occasion as this. His mom's letter assured him that his family loved him and was thinking of him. He felt somewhat reassured, but I knew we were not out of the woods yet.

"You'll get to know these kids," I assured him. "They all started out just like you, feeling nervous about being away from home." I kept watching his face to see if anything I said brought any relief. I couldn't tell for sure. But I kept trying to coax him. I put my hand on his back to let him know that he wasn't in this alone.

"Why don't you go over and get your swimming trunks on," I said. "We can join the others in the pool." He nodded and said that sounded all right.

Things were looking up.

As I played with the kids in the pool, I watched this boy out of the corner of my eye. He began, hesitatingly at first, to participate. He started splashing around in the water a little bit. Before long, he was joining the scramble to the bottom of the pool to grab for the rings I was throwing. That afternoon he got more comfortable with several of the kids, and that boy, who had been on the verge of calling it quits and heading home, ended up having a great experience at camp. I felt as if I had made a difference in this boy's life. Rather than ending his camp adventure unsuccessfully, he got to know other kids with diabetes and learned more about handling his condition himself.

Months later, when I walked into the Christmas party that the American Diabetes Association puts on for the kids, that same boy was crowding around me to say hello, right alongside the others. This time, he had a smile on his face.

Many of these kids have had diabetes since age 2 or 3. Yet they are not self-pitying, nor do they want special treatment from those around them. They simply go on with normal lives. They cheer at football games, play with their friends, worry about getting their homework done—just like other kids. Watching them has helped me adapt to diabetes as part of my life. I have to deal with it; I can't ignore it. But these kids have shown me that diabetes does not have to stand in the way of a normal, satisfying life. Failure or success will be determined by the kind of person I am, not by the fact that my pancreas does not produce insulin.

## Hayes Huddle

After being with these kids for a couple of summer camp sessions as well as at other events the American Diabetes Association scheduled during the year, I started thinking that I would like to do more for these Kansas City area kids with diabetes. A few of them had the opportunity to attend some Chiefs games; some of their families had season tickets. Many of them, though, had never seen a National Football League game.

I worked out an arrangement with the American Diabetes Association and the Chiefs' public relations office to reserve a section of seats in one of the end zones for these kids. My mother suggested the name "Hayes Huddle" for the group; we concluded it was a good fit. I agreed to pay for twenty tickets for each home game and Hayes Huddle T-shirts; Price Chopper, an area grocery store chain and regular Chiefs sponsor, agreed to donate special sack lunches, since these kids with diabetes have to stick close to their diet plan. So since 1990, my personal fan club has cheered me on at every Chiefs home game. Over the railing behind one of the end zones hangs a large banner in their honor. It depicts a red-jerseyed football player wearing number 85. The large black letters on the banner spell: "Hayes Huddle."

Over the years, these kids have become my friends. In any good friendship, the benefits flow both ways. I have had opportunities to give to them, like the boy I helped adjust to summer camp. And they have given to me—like the little girl, and so many others like her, who teach me lessons about courage.

# CHAPTER
## 7

# BUILDING
# SUCCESS

During training camp in Wisconsin in 1991, one of the team doctors brought up a group of kids who were participating in the Special Olympics that week. He asked me to take a few minutes after practice to spend time with them. I agreed.

Coach Schottenheimer pushed us hard that day. For the last few drills, I was visualizing holding my head under the hot shower and relaxing. When he blew the final whistle, I breathed a sigh of relief and headed for the locker room. Before I reached the door, I saw the group of kids standing along the sideline. My first thought was to keep the encounter as brief as possible, then slip on into the locker room.

As I walked over, though, and watched their faces light up, I found myself in less of a hurry. After a few minutes, I began to feel what I always do—that these people, facing significant physical and mental limitations, know about life. They know about giving their best, about overcoming the odds, about living life to its fullest. As we were wrapping up our visit, one of the boys handed me a Special Olympics flag, which I carried back and placed in my locker.

For the rest of the season, that flag reminded me

of that young man who despite the obstacle of his physical and mental limitations was giving his best. As far as I am concerned, that young man is a success.

## Value the Valuable

We need to be careful about how we measure success in our society. It's not just a matter of how much money a person makes, how many times he's on television, or how many people gather in a stadium to watch him perform.

Success is a matter of working hard to be the best person that you can be, no matter how many obstacles stand between you and the goal.

My grandparents showed me a model of success. My grandfather (my dad's father) worked two jobs in Muncie, Ind., to provide for his family of 11 children. But he still found time to teach his children the important lessons at home that laid a solid foundation in their lives. My grandmother (my mom's mother) took pride in being both a good mother and a responsible worker. My grandparents were proud people and were not afraid of hard work. They worked hard at jobs that today might seem less than glamorous. But they conducted their lives with great and beautiful dignity. It was this model of success that influenced my parents and, in turn, my brothers and me.

The day I signed with the Chiefs, or more precisely, the day I deposited the check for my signing bonus, I realized life would be different. In my first couple of years in professional football, the Chiefs paid me more than my parents would earn in their entire careers, my mother as a school teacher and my father as a civil servant in the criminal justice system. But my success, like theirs, will be measured by more than money earned.

While I am certainly grateful for the paychecks, I

have tried to keep a reasonable perspective about the importance of football in society and in my own life. Football is a game. The contests provide an enjoyable diversion for millions of fans each season. But the contribution of other groups, other professions, other workers are of greater value to our society. I have never saved a life on the football field. But nurses and doctors do every day. Football does not teach children to read and write, but teachers invest their entire work lives in molding the minds of those children. It is puzzling to observe the way people value professional athletes, while the most valuable contributions to our society are being made in classrooms, in hospitals, in community youth centers, and other work places less glamorous than the football field.

I'm not sure that it is good for professional athletes to become the primary heroes to a generation of children. Today's kids need heroes in their homes. They need fathers and mothers who invest time in caring and providing for them, talking with them and training them. As a professional athlete, I never want to supplant a parent in the eyes of a child. The parent may not be able to play professional football. But that parent can still be a model of success, a model of what it is to be the best person possible.

Living a successful life means, among other things, hard work. I learned a work ethic in my home. My parents worked us hard around the house with chores and regular responsibilities. My brothers and I swept floors, cleaned bathrooms, cooked meals, cut the grass, and shoveled snow. We knew how to work.

Now, my responsibilities are larger, but the work ethic and the discipline are part of me. Because of my occupation, my responsibility is to remain in the best physical condition possible, to give my best on the football field. Granted, the rewards are good, but they do not come without hard work, discipline, and responsibility.

These same characteristics help me manage my diabetes too. It's hard work to be the doctor of my own body. It takes great discipline to maintain a regular routine of eating, monitoring my blood, and taking medicine. But putting forth the daily effort to manage my diabetes means I can feel good and get my job done on the football field.

# Facing Adversity

When I started school at Iowa, I had a teammate named Tim who had a speech impediment. It was painful to listen to him speak; he had to labor through his stuttering just to make a simple statement. At first we avoided talking with him much; we never wanted to ask him a question. We didn't want to put him on the spot and force him to speak.

But in addition to regular class work and football practice throughout his freshman year, Tim worked hard in a speech therapy program. Tim's speech improved dramatically.

Each year before school started, the football team would have a three-week training camp. Each evening during that camp, Coach Fry would have a player stand up and talk about his goals, his thoughts about the team, and whatever else he had on his mind.

In our sophomore year, Timmy wanted to get up during this camp and make a speech. The whole room was deathly quiet. We were shocked that he wanted to address the entire team and worried about how it would go.

By now, I don't remember a word he said. I only remember that he said a lot of words. He said each of them clearly, with almost no stuttering.

Timmy spoke from his heart and it was powerful.

The room was filled that night with big, tough football players, each one fighting to keep from breaking down in tears in front of his teammates. I had a lump in my throat that night, and I still get a lump in my throat whenever I talk about Timmy.

Here was a guy who wanted to show his friends, his teammates, that he had not only been working to improve himself as a football player, but he also had been working hard to improve himself as a person. He could easily have retreated into an internal world of insecurity. But he faced his condition, he accepted the challenge presented to him, and he overcame it.

That, in my estimation, is success.

## Finding Success

During the journey of my life, I have had the opportunity to meet many people. I have listened to their words and watched their actions. The ones I would consider successful are the ones who have been willing to accept the challenges of life and give their best to meet them.

Of course, everyone will fall short of perfect performance. No one will look back on life and brag about a perfect track record. There is no tragedy in trying and failing, and then trying again. The tragedy is never trying in the first place. If you don't try, you'll never know what you might have been able to accomplish. Regardless of your situation, the only barriers that can stop you from succeeding are the ones you allow to remain in your own path.

One thing you can count on in life is that you will face adversity. Yours may come in a different package than mine. Some have to stare poverty in the face and decide to set aside their excuses and apply themselves to building a successful life. Some must endure tragedy—the loss of a child, a parent, or a spouse—and find a way to pick up the pieces and continue on.

Some, like me, must face a day in a doctor's office when they are told they have a serious disease. The question is not whether adversity will find its way onto the path of our lives. The question is, how will we greet it when it comes? How will we respond? Will we yield to the temptation to use our adversity as an excuse for failure, as a reason to give up, as an explanation for an unfulfilled life?

Or will we have the courage to face the adversity without letting it destroy us? Without lying down and quitting? Of course there will be tough seasons in life, when it will be tough to imagine going on. We don't have to be too proud to accept help during those times. But over the long haul, we have to face the adversity, absorb its blows like the crushing block of a defensive tackle, then get up and continue going forward.

I have had my dose of adversity. Much of mine has come from a tiny little organ tucked inside my midsection that doesn't work properly. For some reason, it doesn't produce insulin. Diabetes is a serious disease, a vigilant opponent that stalks me continually, looking for a chink in my armor of protection. With proper eating and exercise, and monitoring and medicine, I can control it reasonably well. But if I let down my defense against this deadly opponent, it can wreak havoc in my body. It can cost me a leg or my eyesight. It can beat up my heart and tear down my kidneys. And at any time, diabetes could cost me my life.

While the disease is serious, and its threat should never be underestimated, I have the benefits of living in a day of advanced medical care and increased understanding about controlling the disease. Good management of my diabetes keeps the window of opportunity open for me to live a full and satisfying life. But that window doesn't stay open by itself. I have to work to keep it open.

The typical athlete mentality about health is a dangerous one, especially for me. Athletes tend to consider themselves invincible. Because he's big, he's strong, and he works out regularly, he thinks it will take a lot to knock him down. He is invincible, he thinks. But I'll be in serious trouble if I let that attitude make much headway in my life.

I know I am not invincible. Diabetes is a relentless opponent. But I have stared that opponent in the face; I have been stubborn enough not to let diabetes stop me from striving to reach my goals on and off the field. If diabetes is part of your dose of adversity, then I encourage you to face it courageously and find ways to continue your pursuit of a satisfying and successful life. That, of course, doesn't necessarily mean becoming a professional football player. It means being the best person you can be, contributing what you have to give to society, looking for opportunities to help other people, accepting the responsibilities that come with becoming an individual human being.

It may not be diabetes that threatens to interfere with your pursuit of a full life. You may have walked into a doctor's office and come out with your ears resounding to the diagnosis of cancer, lung disease, multiple sclerosis, or muscular dystrophy. Or you may have a child, or a parent, or a close friend who has heard equally devastating news from a doctor.

Your adversity may have nothing to do with health. Broken relationships, abuse, unemployment, and deep disappointments can also tackle you on the path your life follows.

But adversity does not have to cause you to fail. If you can look adversity in the face, absorb its blows, and find a way to keep running downfield toward your goal, then you, my friend, have discovered success. In my book, you have reason to hold your head high. You have reason to celebrate your accomplishments, for you have met the challenge that your life has presented. You have joined the ranks of those who have overcome adversity and touched success.

# ABOUT THE AMERICAN DIABETES ASSOCIATION

The American Diabetes Association (ADA) is the nation's leading voluntary health organization dedicated to improving the well-being of all people affected by diabetes. Equally important is its unceasing support for research to prevent and cure this chronic disease that affects some 13 million Americans. The Association carries out this important mission through the efforts of thousands of volunteers working at state affiliates and local chapters in more than 800 communities throughout the United States.

Membership in the American Diabetes Association puts you in contact with a network of more than 270,000 caring people throughout the country. Affiliates and chapters offer support groups, educational programs, counseling, and other special services. Membership also brings twelve issues of the lively patient education magazine, *Diabetes Forecast*.

In addition, the Association publishes an array of materials for every age group on topics important not just to the individual with diabetes, but to the entire family. Considerable effort is also devoted to educating health-care professionals and building public awareness about diabetes. To receive a free copy of the Healthy Living Catalog, call 1-800-232-3472, ext. 363.

Information on American Diabetes Association memberships and programs is available through the state affiliates (listed in the white pages of the telephone book) or through the American Diabetes Association, 1660 Duke Street, Alexandria, VA 22314; 1-800-232-3472, ext. 343.

# ABOUT DIABETES

### *What Is Diabetes?*

Diabetes mellitus is a chronic disease in which the body does not produce or respond to insulin. Insulin is a hormone, produced by the pancreas, that helps the body metabolize the sugar glucose. When insulin is absent or ineffective, high levels of glucose appear in the blood. High blood glucose levels can lead to both short-term and long-term complications.

### *What Are the Major Types of Diabetes?*

There are two major types of diabetes mellitus: insulin-dependent diabetes mellitus (IDDM, also called type I) and non-insulin-dependent diabetes mellitus (NIDDM, also called type II). Another type of diabetes is gestational diabetes mellitus, a term used to describe impaired glucose tolerance that has its onset or is first detected during pregnancy.

### *How Is Diabetes Treated?*

Diabetes therapy is geared toward controlling high blood glucose levels (hyperglycemia) and preventing diabetes complications. For IDDM, treatment consists of insulin injections and diet/exercise therapy. For NIDDM, treatment may include insulin injections or oral agents to lower blood glucose, diet therapy, a weight-reduction program for patients who are overweight, and a program of exercise. Monitoring of blood glucose—by both the person with diabetes and the physician—is an important adjunct to the care of both forms of diabetes.

### *How Many People in the United States Have Diabetes?*

Counting both diagnosed and undiagnosed diabetes, as many as 13 million people, or 5.2 percent of the U.S. population, have diabetes. Although this estimate is for diabetes of all types, almost 98 percent of people older than 20 with diabetes have NIDDM.

### *How Many Children Have Diabetes?*

There are about 120,000 children with IDDM in the United States. Peak incidence is around 10 to 12 years old in girls and 12 to 14 years old in boys.

### *Who Is Most Likely to Get Diabetes?*

Diabetes prevalence increases with increasing age, with about half of all cases in people older than 55. Nearly 17 percent of the U.S. white population 65 to 74 years old has diabetes. The prevalence of diabetes tends to be slightly higher in women than in men, especially in black Americans.

### *Does Diabetes Occur More Often in Minorities?*

Yes. NIDDM tends to be more common in minority populations than in whites. Overall, the prevalence of diabetes is about 30 percent higher in blacks than in whites. By ages 65 to 74, 25 percent of blacks and more than 33 percent of Hispanics have diabetes, compared with 17 percent of whites. In one study, Mexican Americans were nearly three times as likely to develop NIDDM as non-Hispanic whites living in the same area.

## *How Many New Cases of Diabetes Will There Be This Year?*

More than 650,000 new cases of diabetes are diagnosed each year. The majority of these people have NIDDM. The incidence of diabetes has increased slightly during the 1980s, primarily in the older age groups and in women.

## *How Serious Is Diabetes?*

Very serious. Diabetes mellitus is the seventh-leading cause of death and the fourth-leading cause of death by disease in the United States. Mortality caused by diabetes represents about 1.8 percent of total U.S. mortality. Each year, about 160,000 people die from diabetes and its complications. But these statistics greatly underestimate the true mortality due to diabetes because it is well known that diabetes is underreported on death certificates. The total cost of diabetes in the United States is staggering: more than $90 billion per year.

### *How Common Are Complications of Diabetes?*

Studies have shown that people with diabetes are four times as likely to die from heart disease as people who don't have diabetes. They are four times as likely to have blockages of arteries in the legs and feet (peripheral arterial disease). Stroke is also more common in people with diabetes. Stroke occurs about two times more frequently in people with diabetes than in people without diabetes. Diabetic eye disease (retinopathy) is also common; by 5 years after the diagnosis of diabetes, retinopathy is present in 14 percent of younger-onset (before 30 years of age) people with diabetes and 40 percent of older-onset insulin-taking people with diabetes. Diabetic kidney disease (nephropathy) occurs in 34 percent of IDDM and 19 percent of NIDDM patients after 15 years with the disease. Nerve complications (neuropathy) are present at diagnosis in about 8 percent of people with diabetes; 25 years after diagnosis, at least half of all affected people have developed neuropathy.

### *How Serious Are the Complications of Diabetes?*

In the United States, diabetes is responsible for about 12,000 cases of legal blindness each year, making it a leading cause of new cases of blindness in adults 25 to 74 years old. Kidney disease (diabetic nepropathy) may progress to end-stage renal disease (ESRD) and death. Thirty-two percent of new cases of ESRD—more than 13,000 cases each year—are attributable to diabetes. Diabetic neuropathy can lead to loss of sensation in feet and legs, amputation, silent myocardial infarction, and sudden death.

## Can Diabetes and Its Complications Be Prevented?

It is likely that the complications of diabetes can be greatly reduced in severity, if not prevented, if people with diabetes control obesity, reduce cholesterol levels, exercise, stop smoking, and improve control of blood glucose levels. Early identification and treatment of diabetes complications are also essential for limiting their severity and improving quality of life. A recent evaluation of national data concluded that half of NIDDM cases and at least half of most major complications could be prevented by appropriate education and intervention programs.

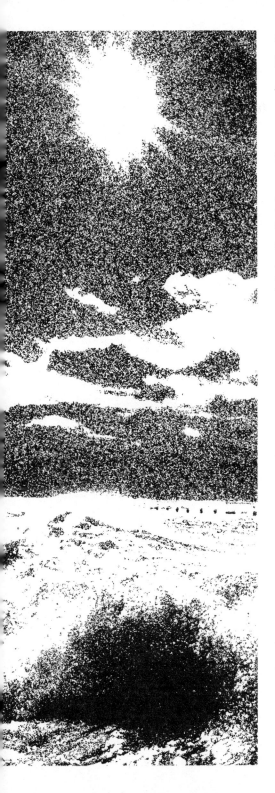

# Sharing the Spirit

Many personal stories of living with diabetes offer messages of enlightenment and hope. For the millions of people who have diabetes, hearing such stories may inspire encouragement to develop a healthier outlook about the changes this disease has brought to their lives. Miles Inc., marketer of the GLUCOMETER ELITE™ Diabetes Care System, is grateful for the opportunity to help share the spirit of successful living with diabetes through its sponsorship of this book.

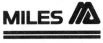

**MILES**

**Diagnostics Division**